f

NEUROPSYCHOLOGY AND AGING
Definitions, Explanations and
Practical Approaches

NEUROPSYCHOLOGY AND AGING

Definitions, Explanations and Practical Approaches

Edited by Una Holden

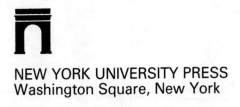

NEW YORK UNIVERSITY PRESS
Washington Square, New York

First published in the USA in 1988 by
New York University Press
Washington Square, New York NY 10003

© 1988 Una Holden

LIBRARY OF CONGRESS
Library of Congress Cataloging-in-Publication Data
Neuropsychology and aging : definitions, explanations and practical
    approaches / edited by Una Holden.
        p.   cm.
    Includes bibliographies and index.
    ISBN 0-8147-3459-6
    1. Geriatric neuropsychiatry.   2. Clinical neuropsychology.
    3. Senile dementia — Diagnosis.   4. Brain damage — Diagnosis.
    I. Holden, Una P.
    [DNLM: 1. Nervous System Diseases — in old age.
    2. Neuropsychology — in old age.   WL 103 N49352]
    RC451.4.A5N47   1988
    618.97'689 — dc19
    DNLM/DLC
    for Library of Congress   88-22424
                                                     CIP

Printed and bound in Great Britain

To Cormac, Triona, Niall, Niamh, Angus, Mhairi, and Ben

Contents

Contributors

Jeffrey L. Cummings, MD. Director, Neurobehavioral Unit, West Los Angeles Veterans Administration Medical Center (Brentwood Division) and Department of Neurology and Department of Psychiatry and Behavioral Sciences, University of California, Los Angeles School of Medicine, Los Angeles, California, USA.

Una Holden (now Holden-Cosgrove). Principal Clinical Psychologist, Garlands Hospital, Carlisle, England. Previously Chief Clinical Tutor and Senior Lecturer, Plymouth; now Freelance Consultant Clinical Psychologist, Ironmacannie Mill, Balmaclellan, Castle Douglas, Kirkcudbrightshire, Scotland.

Judith Aharon Peretz, MD. Neurobehavioral Unit, West Los Angeles Veterans Administration Medical Center (Brentwood Division) and Department of Neurology, University of California, Los Angeles School of Medicine, Los Angeles, California, USA.

Ian Thompson, PhD. Previously National College of Speech Sciences, London; now Department of Speech Pathology, Prince Henry's Hospital, St Kilda Road, Melbourne, Victoria 3004, Australia.

Preface

For many days my brain
Worked with a dim and undetermined sense
Of unknown modes of being (Wordsworth)

Over the years it has become increasingly apparent that those working with elderly people are facing added difficulties due to the lack of understanding of behaviours related to damage of brain function. Originally this book was intended to provide basic information for those outside the medical and psychological professions who had no knowledge of neuropsychology. At present such knowledge is limited to the few who specialise in the field, and for whom most books on the subject are written. Manuals concerning the rehabilitation of adults and children are beginning to appear, but the wide range of involved staff has been forgotten and there is barely a mention of elderly people's problems. Gerontology is a new science, but the volume of literature on ageing processes is growing so it is now possible to find guidance on treatment and management of specific problems. However, very little attention has been paid to the influence of neuropsychological factors. This omission has led to mistakes in goal-setting, unsatisfactory interventions and rehabilitation schemes.

After some consideration the aims of this volume have been extended to include the more experienced professionals by adding more detailed and particular subjects. As the application of neuropsychological approaches with elderly patients or clients is still in its infancy, even rethinking basic concepts can lead to new ideas and different avenues which could improve the service offered to the older generation.

It is hoped that the gaps in the knowledge and practice of neuropsychology will be filled in — even a little — by these pages which are intended to clarify some of the terms, provide explanations, suggestions for simple and realistic assessments and outline some practical approaches to fairly common problems. To attempt to supply clear-cut answers at this stage in the development of the subject of neuropsychology of ageing is unrealistic. Though many answers can be supplied by applying common sense to the growing volume of knowledge, there is still so much to learn and a great demand for more research.

There is already available enough information to encourage awareness, reconsider management and interventions and their degree of value to the individual, as well as a need to question assumptions and incomplete assessments.

Neuropsychology is the study of behaviour directly related to brain function. Although most people accept that psychological factors play an important role in influencing behaviour the influence of neuropsychological factors is rarely considered. Certain observed reactions, or lack of reactions, may be as a result of damage to part of the brain rather than to personality moods, attitudes or affective disorders. To assume that certain behaviours have such simple explanations could well obscure the real problems and needs. Neuropsychology is not a new science; in fact man was aware of brain function in, at least, the seventeenth century BC. The papyrus on which accounts of head injury were written could date from 3000 BC. Hippocrates, Aristotle, Galen and others from ancient times developed theories about the function and importance of the brain. Gall, amongst others, produced phrenological maps which can still be seen in libraries. The late nineteenth century produced some of the classical contributors — Paul Broca and Carl Wernicke — who were followed in recent years by such great scientists as Aleksandr Romanovitch Luria. Luria was one of the foremost workers in restoration of function, and his practical applications have inspired others to search for further appropriate methods of rehabilitation.

The role of a neuropsychologist includes:

1. assisting in diagnosis;
2. providing relevant assessment tools and methods;
3. finding methods to distinguish organic damage from functional states;
4. monitoring change;
5. identifying precipitants, e.g. effects of light on epilepsy;
6. predicting outcome;
7. assisting in the isolation and identification of new systems or pathways, syndromes or other aspects of brain-related behaviour;
8. developing and assisting in rehabilitation and restoration of function programmes;
9. counselling and providing support for families of clients;
10. research.

The topics to be discussed in this book will include some of the more recent research as well as basic concepts. The first chapter, while providing definitions and explanations of the soft signs, also considers the various interpretations of observed behaviours and the false conclusions that can be reached. Chapter 2 focuses on simple assessment and lists the more obvious signs to be identified. It provides a screening procedure and stresses the importance of watching and listening in the search for explanations. Confusion and dementia are the subjects of Chapter 3. Recent research is included in an argument against the existence of a specific disease process called 'senile dementia'.

Subcortical dementias have only been recognised within the past ten years or so, and are still unknown to many professionals, including some physicians. Drs Cummings and Peretz from Los Angeles provide a very full overview of a subject that should be appreciated by all concerned with the care of elderly people, as well as adult neurological patients. This detailed account should help to increase recognition and understanding of conditions which are too often overlooked in hospital wards and outpatient clinics, and provide guidelines for treatment and management programmes.

Communication changes — Chapter 5 — is contributed by Dr Ian Thompson from Melbourne, who provides a valuable update on language research. He stresses the differences between normal age changes and those brought about by specific disease processes, the urgency of proper identification of disorders for the sake of the client and the differences between specific damage and that caused by Alzheimer's disease. An overview of treatment programmes is also included.

Head injury is a matter of public concern, yet elderly head-injured people are often 'written off' and denied the understanding and support that they require. Research is sparse and knowledge limited. Chapter 6 attempts to highlight some of the problems and possible approaches to rehabilitation. The two final chapters are concerned with treatment and possible approaches to particular impairments. Hyperventilation, for instance, is a common complaint which is often overlooked and not even included in DSM III; there are many papers on the subject, but, once again, the elderly are neglected.

As far as possible case studies have been included to illustrate the problem, variations from person to person or the programmes that were used to help an individual. If this book does no more than provoke readers to challenge the arguments and practical suggestions by open discussion or further research then it will have achieved its purpose. If in the process of this staff members begin to question conclusions on observed behaviour, the goals that are set, the omission of neuropsychological factors in assessments and if more training courses include the subject then, inevitably, elderly people will receive a better service.

The editor would like to express her thanks to the contributors whose chapters add to the slowly expanding store of well-researched information and who have given encouragement to those who for so long have worked in an atmosphere of 'no hope' or 'no outside interest'. She would also like to express her appreciation of Miss Sheena Dumpe's patience, and the long hours she spent in preparing this manuscript.

1

Recognising the Problems

Una Holden

At all ages human behaviour can be misinterpreted. We are all familiar with the problems faced in a doctor's surgery where both patient and physician struggle to get their messages across to each other. The patient attempts to explain the aches, pains and feelings in a meaningful manner, and the doctor tries to make sense of all the various symptoms in order to arrive at a correct diagnosis. Frequently both are frustrated by a perceived lack of understanding on the part of the other. Such a situation occurs every day in most interpersonal contacts. The stress is placed wrongly on a word, a gesture is misunderstood, someone deep in thought apparently ignores an acquaintance, a work situation appears threatening when it is only reflecting anxiety and a husband and wife relationship is put under duress because one or other partner is tired. These upsets in personal relationships are commonplace and, to a degree, easy to appreciate. However, there are specific behaviours for which there does not appear to be a reasonable explanation, and even the professionals are liable to error.

Mankind automatically explains his perceptions according to his experience, expectations, ability and knowledge. As all of these are essentially finite, errors frequently occur. People rarely stop to think, to examine the facts or to make further enquiry. Everyone is in a rush and too busy to pause. To spend valuable time on searching for alternatives interferes in the progress of work or interests and is regarded as a nuisance, or too demanding. No-one is genuinely willing to admit to ignorance so when an unusual situation arises an answer has to be found which will satisfy speculation without too much pressure on time.

Odd behaviour is viewed with some discomforture and often

a pejorative remark will be used to dismiss the problem. However, there are many explanations for odd behaviour, including:

The person is really odd — idiosyncratic, or the local 'character'.

There is a medical reason — delirium, amnesia, deafness, blindness.

The problem is physiologically based — malnutrition, drug-induced, narcolepsy, etc.

Psychiatric disturbance could be present.

The unfortunate person has poor social skills.

He or she has had a head injury.

There could be a neuropsychological explanation.

Therapists are constantly faced with the difficulties of handling negative approaches to life. Cognitive therapy highlights the classical situation by using as an example 'Mrs Jones', who is convinced that her neighbour does not like her because she walked straight past her in the street. When other explanations of the 'dislike' are offered, 'Mrs Jones' is persuaded to look again. Her neighbour could have visual difficulties, she could have been deep in thought, worrying, or even thinking happily about a pleasant experience. Hopefully one of these suggestions proves correct, so the client can begin to develop a more positive view of herself and her life. Sometimes the original, negative perception proves to be correct and the unfortunate therapist is faced with another problem!

It is surprising how rarely pejorative statements or erroneous explanations are challenged. Behaviour of those with head injury or neurological deficits, and that of old people, is invariably labelled, yet there are few who would question that label. Case notes contain words such as 'aggressive', 'unmotivated' and 'violent', but the reason for the use of such strong words is never investigated. 'Incontinent' could mean that the person could not find the toilet and was unable to wait any longer. 'Aggression' could reflect someone's anger at being sat next to a patient who consistently spat, swore and interfered. 'Violent' could mean that a peacefully sleeping patient was suddenly approached from behind and laid hold of without warning in order that a wound could be dressed. The possibility that the 'violent' response might be a purely defensive one is rarely considered. When reasons or preceding events are not recorded the omissions give a false perspective which can lead to the permanent attachment of pejorative labels.

Neuropsychological factors are not understood by the general public. Care staff too may be ignorant of them. To some nurses the words may be familiar, but the complicated definitions remain vague. Unfortunately too many of the other professionals are equally unsure on the subject, with the result that appropriate treatment and understanding are not always provided. This occurs with all age groups, particularly with head injuries and regularly so with the over-60s.

Geriatric wards and residential homes daily provide examples of misinterpreted behaviours and overlooked problems because of ignorance of their possible implications. Table 1.1 offers examples of the commoner behaviours and the possible conclusions drawn by staff and other observers. It is understandable if relatives of clients living at home make such assumptions, particularly when any source of support is unable to suggest alternative explanations. There are many more situations than those in Table 1.1 and, obviously many more explanations. Where there is genuine lack of available knowledge the observer can be forgiven for the misinterpretations. Generally, even when information can be obtained it proves easier to jump to conclusions. If a good service is to be offered

Table 1.1: Examples of common behaviour and explanations

Behaviour observed	Explanation offered
Walking into things.	Forgetful. Blind.
Drops things, lacks dexterity.	Clumsy.
Gets into someone else's bed.	Over-sexed.
Complains of an assault.	Litigation minded.
Very slow. No response.	Unco-operative. Losing his/her mind.
Eats very little.	Anorexic. Apathetic.
Will not dress.	Difficult. Unmotivated.
Does not recognise faces, or objects.	Blind. Apathetic.
Dizzy spells. Falling. Fainting. Gasping for breath.	Epileptic. Attention-seeking.
Sings beautifully but does not talk.	Lazy. Attention-seeking. Unco-operative.
Says nothing meaningful; uses funny words or phrases.	Totally deteriorated.
Cries or laughs inappropriately.	Very sad. Upset by past. Upset by present state.
Forgets to give a message.	Senile.

to those in need all available information should be carefully sought and included in initial examinations. To set goals for any client without covering all known possibilities is to court disaster. Staff training should include neuropsychology which would then considerably lessen the error factor. Many attempts have been made to show how neuropsychological deficits can cause specific problems (e.g. Benson, 1979; Albert, 1981; Holden and Woods, 1988), but observers often fail to make the connection between the behaviour they see and the possibility of specific brain damage. Admittedly, the lack of convincing published evidence of success of neuropsychological rehabilitative methods could have cast doubt as to the value of including neuropsychology in training (Miller, 1984). It is only a matter of time before this is available. Furthermore it is no excuse for neglecting an important possible explanation for 'odd' behaviour.

TERMINOLOGY

For a detailed account of neuropsychology there are a number of relevant textbooks available (e.g. Hecaen and Albert, 1978; Walsh, 1987). The correct meaning of the prefix 'A' implies 'lack of' or 'without', and the prefix 'dys' implies 'damaged' or 'disordered'. In current practice the prefixes are used more loosely, so that either can indicate the presence of damage, usually acquired.

Aphasia

Aphasia is a disturbance of language and includes speech, reading, writing and calculations. Generally it refers to speech, but it should include all other forms of language. Language is associated with the dominant hemisphere — usually left — and the relevant centres and systems therein.

Agraphia. Agraphia, or dysgraphia, refers to a disturbance of writing and can vary in severity from a total inability to write to peculiar spelling, odd ways of forming letters or even small errors such as repeated or omitted letters or words. This is not due to a disability of the hand, arm or muscles, or to a lack of knowledge of how to write.

4

Alexia.   Alexia, or dyslexia, usually implies that there are reading difficulties. At present there is some controversy about the use of this term, but the argument is irrelevant in this context. If a person has difficulty in reading or in making sense of the written word some form of alexia is present.

Acalculia.   Refers to the problems with mathematics. Adding up, recognising or writing numbers, calculating the cost of shopping, as well as handling more complicated mathematical problems that once were straightforward, are all to be considered under this heading.

Of course, the client's educational background must be taken into account with all of these language disorders. Someone who never learned to read, write or to add cannot be expected to demonstrate such skills, and could prove a difficult client to assess for language disabilities.

Speech disorders are most often noted after a person has suffered a stroke, though there are a number of other causes of such impairments.

Dysarthria.   This is often mistaken for an aphasia. It is frequently defined as imperfect articulation, as the speech sounds so indistinct. However, there is much more involved than articulation. Impairments may be present in respiration, phonation, resonance, volume, rate, voice quality, intonation or rhythm. The person has no problems with word finding, sentence construction, expression of thoughts or any of the difficulties associated with a true aphasia, just with actual oral communication. To the listener the person sounds strange, guttural, drunk, foreign or very quietly spoken. This dysarthria is due to a lesion in the upper or lower motor neurones, the basal ganglia or in the cerebellum, which results in weakness, paralysis or inco-ordination of the muscles and mechanisms associated with the larynx, pharynx or tongue. It is important to note the differences between language and speech:

1. *Language*
   Sounds, symbols, gestures; a learned and ordered system.
2. *Speech*
   Actual production of words and the use of all the physical components to do so.

5

Linguistics is the transmission of messages in one particular language.

Language has four components:

sounds: phonology/phonics;
lexical system: vocabulary and gesture;
grammar: syntax;
meaning: semantic system.

Several words are used to describe the different aspects of speech:

Phonation: the basic system of speech necessary for the production of words.
Articulation: actual production of speech.
Phonemes: each sound. These sounds must be strung together to obtain meaning.
Prosody: melodious aspect of speech which adds and clarifies meaning.

The process of speech requires that thought is sorted out in the Wernicke's area, which is usually in the left dominant hemisphere involving the posterior part of the superior temporal gyrus (approximately where the left temporal lobe joins into the frontal and parietal lobes). Here meanings are found, responses or ideas are made sensible, pictorial or written material is converted into verbal components, answers are found to auditory input and then transmitted (usually via the angular gyrus) to Broca's area in the posterior part of the frontal lobes (inferior frontal convolution). Providing that there is no malfunction all the necessary expressive components are added in Broca's, the motor cortex is stimulated and speech is produced. This is greatly simplifying the process, but is in essence what happens. Although man has much to learn about brain function, and even language processes are still not fully researched, speechlessness, as a result of brain damage to certain areas, has been recognised since 3000 BC. Paul Broca in the mid-nineteenth century contributed enormously to the theories of localisation of function, and it was he who put forward the idea that speech was localised in the left hemisphere. About twelve years later Carl Wernicke added more detail to these contributions and delineated the posterior part of the superior temporal gyrus (where the left temporal lobe connects with the frontal and parietal lobes) as the area concerned with comprehension.

Disorders of speech are generally divided into two types:

1. *Broca's aphasia.* Also called expressive, non-fluent, motor. Usual area concerned: Left dominant hemisphere — Third Frontal convolution.
2. *Wernicke's aphasia.* Also called receptive, fluent, sensory. Usual area concerned: Left dominant hemisphere — Posterior part of the superior temporal gyrus.

The features of *Broca's aphasia* are:

No real comprehension problems.

Anomia (word-finding problems).

Phonemes are mixed up, e.g. p for b, pelsil for pencil.

Automatic speech is good.

Telegraphic agrammatism — omitting verbs, prefixes etc. — only using key words.

Reading and writing is usually impaired.

As there is often insight frustration is common – can become angry or weepy.

Speech is often awkward, hesitant and sparse.

Some of the articulatory difficulties could be due to dyspraxia.

Can name, but cannot repeat. As comprehension is preserved can read, but not out loud.

Automatic phrases may be the only speech, e.g. 'Five, five five'. 'I don't know what to say'. 'Hello/Goodbye'.

Probably about 60–70 per cent of aphasics are of this type.

The main features of *Wernicke's aphasia* are:

As there is usually no motor deficit, speech will flow.

As often auditory comprehension is damaged information received is meaningless. Therefore others are seen as crazy, or as talking rubbish.

Articulation is normal, but the person is paraphasic — uses the wrong word order in sentences, or the wrong word, e.g. mother instead of wife.

Jargon, neologisms, and meaningless verbalisations are typical.

7

Rhythm, stress and intonation are normal.

Anomia (word-finding problems), circumlocution, perseveration and echolalia all occur.

Insight is often lacking.

May look and sound normal.

Behaviour — social responses are perfectly good. Can understand expression and gesture so can pick up social cues.

May laugh loudly and inappropriately — or weep, but rarely
inappropriately.

Could be apraxic.

Writing and reading are usually impaired.

The main areas concerned with Wernicke's aphasia are in the
dominant hemisphere — where the left temporal lobe connects
with the frontal and parietal lobes (the posterior part of the
superior temporal gyrus).

A more detailed account of the aphasias will be found in
Chapter 5. Here it is important to stress that speech and other
language disorders vary from person to person. Some patients
are especially affected, whilst others only appear to hesitate, to
be slow or not very agile mentally. It is possible for a person to
have both Broca's and Wernicke's, one usually more
pronounced than the other. Contact with other people can be
profoundly disturbed, particularly when good oral communication is impossible or when the problems are so great that the
person appears to be psychotic. Mildly impaired people can
become increasingly anxious in company as they are aware of
their errors and hesitations, and may well be so embarrassed
and frustrated by them that they avoid the social scene entirely
and increase their difficulties through lack of practice and
limited success.

The complications that are often associated, e.g. agraphia,
acalculia, can assist the diagnosis and help to localise a lesion, so
all variations in individual language problems should be
carefully recorded.

Apraxia

This refers to a series of movement disorders. It implies an
impairment of voluntary and purposeful movements which is
not caused by limb, muscle, or mechanism weakness or defect,

nor is it due to lack of comprehension. The person is quite capable of performing the actions and will do so automatically. The individual fully appreciates what to do, but the moment the movement comes under conscious control begins to experience difficulties. The organisation and co-ordination of thought and appropriate action are not operating effectively. The motor mechanic who has taken cars apart and put them back together for many years begins to replace a new part and suddenly finds that he cannot work out what goes where. The lady who has won prizes for her knitting suddenly finds she cannot make a purl stitch. The disorder is quite common, but is frequently misinterpreted.

The principal forms of apraxia are: dressing, ideomotor, ideational, constructional, buccofacial.

Ideomotor apraxia

Here the person is unable to perform a simple, single gesture. Automatically he or she will wave 'goodbye', pick up something or make some often-used gesture. The moment attention is drawn to such an action the ability to perform it appears to vanish. A Catholic will regularly make the sign of the cross in prayer; when asked to make this sign the person will not know where to start. Understanding is present but the memory for the pattern of performance has been lost in some way. Response by imitation appears to be at a better level. Behavioural responses vary from client to client, e.g. there may be many movements or none at all in attempting tasks.

Ideational apraxia

Here the individual is incapable of carrying out a complex task involving movement. Order and sequence are lost once the act is under voluntary control, and a task which can easily be performed without any thought becomes a traumatic experience and completely disordered. In ideomotor apraxia the plan or engram is preserved but the overall plan and correct sequence is lost. Understanding is present, the person knows what is to be done, but cannot get gestures in the right order. The classical example is to ask the person to take a match from a box, strike it and light a candle. The instructions are understood, the individual is a smoker and lights matches regularly throughout the day, but when asked to do so becomes thoroughly mixed up. The matches drop on the floor, the candle can be rubbed on the box — a total chaos of matches, pieces of box and bits of candle can be the result. As with ideomotor apraxia patients behavioural responses vary. The patient may stop trying after the first error, may make a different action altogether, or may add more and more actions which confuse the response even further. Sometimes imitation appears to be more successful. In acute cases the observer will note that the client's hands resemble a bunch of bananas, with the fingers all stiffly bent. The person is unable to loosen them and all movements of the hand and arm look rigid and even choreiform. When not trying to carry out a set task the hands, arms and movements look quite normal.

Arguments continue over the relationship of ideomotor and ideational apraxia to each other; there are equal differences of opinion about location of lesions and the extent of damage. Though both are often associated with the parietal lobes, different researchers suggest other areas, bilaterality or no localisation at all. Luria felt that different parts of the brain had different roles to play in voluntary control. Such arguments, and more detailed discussion of the apraxias, can be obtained from textbooks on neuropsychology. Here it is more important to stress the need to be aware of the apraxias, to test for them and to take them into account both in rehabilitation programmes and in the understanding of an individual's behaviour.

Constructional apraxia

The presence of constructional apraxia is not easy to establish simply by observation. It may be suggested by apparent difficulties with manipulating things spatially, e.g. assembling mechanisms or objects, even putting jigsaws together. To obtain as much information about its nature as possible some tests should be employed. Often the patient cannot put the parts together in order to complete the whole; on other occasions no parts are correctly joined or constructed. Right hemisphere damage to the parietal or temporoparietal lobes produces visuospatial impairments in which a model does not help, and in fact increases the person's difficulties. When damage occurs in the left parietal or temporoparietal lobes models or cues can help the person to complete the tasks. For instance, if using Block Design patterns the pictures can be of assistance to those with left hemisphere damage so that, at least up to a point, the cubes can be correctly placed to achieve the pattern on the picture. In case of the person with right hemisphere damage the cubes will not be joined together, or will be spread in a straight line or even built into towers with no resemblance to the picture whatsoever. Providing cues for people with non-dominant damage only adds to the confusion.

Present theory suggests a motor defect as a result of left hemisphere lesions, so there is an inability to establish a programme for the right action, and in the case of right hemisphere damage there is a defect in a person's ability to perceive spatial relationships.

Dressing apraxia

This appears to be related to lesions in the non-dominant parietal and occipital areas. In most cases the almost automatic system for dressing oneself has been lost. The relationship of clothes to person is not apparent. True dressing apraxia appears to be separate from one-sided neglect where the person dresses one side of the body but not the other. Dressing apraxia is bilateral and can also be associated with a figure–ground disturbance so that clothes and the area on which they lie cannot be dissociated from each other. This is another visuospatial defect and the degree of deficit varies from person to person. Not all those who have problems with dressing have this form of apraxia, but it is a fairly common problem and should be considered when such difficulties are observed. The engram, or mental plan of dressing, has been lost and the right gesture cannot be found to associate those clothes with the body. Ability to rotate objects in space can also be impaired.

Buccofacial and other apraxias

There are a number of other types of apraxia — whole-body, gait disturbances, loss of ability to sing, whistle or hum, other effects on language and even the buccofacial loss of voluntary movement of the tongue, mouth and other parts of the face. The patient chews, smiles, blows, sucks and sticks out his or her tongue with ease until requested to perform that action. The abilities to wink, raise eyebrows and wiggle the nose are also lost under voluntary direction. Apraxia for speech is a fairly frequent referral for speech therapists.

Agnosia

This is an inability to recognise sensory perceptions which is not

11

due to a defect in the sensory system concerned, ignorance of the nature of the object, the sound, taste, smell or feel, to defective intelligence or to confusion.

This condition is infrequently identified, almost impossible to observe and the subject of much neuropsychological study. The visual form is the commonest.

Visual or object agnosia

This is not only an inability to name or demonstrate the use of an object without touching it, but also a total lack of recognition of the object's meaning or character. The person does not even remember ever seeing anything like it before.

Frequently the problem is misinterpreted as being related to language or visual memory disorders. However, if another sense is introduced recognition is almost immediate. A simple test is to ask the patient to identify, by sight alone, a lipstick case. The shape, colour and perhaps the idea that it is a container will be the response. Once able to handle it and to use other senses recognition is usually immediate. The condition is rare, and as such provokes much argument as to location of the lesion and the true nature of the condition. The right occipital region is frequently mentioned; some authors suggest lesions are in the left occipital area and the splenium, others consider it to be a visuoverbal disconnection syndrome. Whatever its location it is associated with strokes, tumours, head injuries and dementia-related states. Its presence has implications for management programmes.

Two other rare and interesting variations of visual agnosia are prosopagnosia and simultanagnosia.

Prosopagnosia. This is an inability to recognise familiar faces, including the person's own face at times. Relatives can be disturbed by being regarded as a stranger or as a parent instead of a spouse. It is not unknown for a man to accuse his wife of infidelity because he keeps seeing a strange man in the mirror. The same problem is equally common with women. Sometimes this disability is the only presenting problem; sometimes it is one of many. Lesions appear to be related to the right occipital area, but many factors should be considered, as the explanation or real difficulty will vary from individual to individual.

Simultanagnosia. This is an inability to see a whole configuration as each little part of that whole has to be considered first — the person can only see one little bit at a time. The problem is one of synthesis. A still picture cannot be seen as a whole but each tiny part of it will be clearly identified. Similarly a series of moving pictures will prove meaningless but one of the still pictures will make sense. Pictures presented on complicated backgrounds or obscured in some way will cause great confusion and highlight the disability. There appear to be similar difficulties with reading words, which are often seen one letter at a time. Once again, although the occipital lobe appears to be involved, there could be a related language disorder and involvement of several systems rather than a particular location.

Auditory agnosia

This very rare state is demonstrated when a person fails to recognise either speech or sound, or even both. To the afflicted person speech may sound like an unfamiliar foreign language or nonsense talk. Surprisingly, when others slow down their speech the person has no difficulty in understanding the conversation. Problems in identifying unseen noises can be associated with this, or may occur alone. There are obvious dangers for the person with auditory agnosia for sound — honking horns, other sounds indicating warning or danger may prove meaningless unless the person can see from whence they come. Deafness as well as blindness must be excluded before concluding any agnosic state is present.

Spatial agnosia

This is simply an inability to find the way around even familiar places — a disorientation for space. The person may be able to recognise familiar objects but has problems even in identifying the rooms in his or her own home and 'forgets' where things are kept. Maps can also prove meaningless. A flight navigator after sustaining a moderately severe stroke found that he was no longer able to make any sense of his charts, and was considerably relieved to find that as he recovered this ability returned. It is not unusual to find a driver who, whilst on holiday in a strange area, develops some impairment and is no longer capable of following a correct route. Strokes, head injuries, tumours and dementia-related states amongst other disorders are capable of producing this unwelcome state. Loss of topographical memory, visual field defects, difficulties with three

13

dimensions and the manipulation of objects spatially are only some of the difficulties that are considered to fall under this heading. Obviously the right hemisphere and the occipital lobes are much favoured as the site of lesions, but other parts of the brain — particularly the frontal lobes — must be considered in the individual case.

Colour agnosia.　　This is an important indicator of damage in the occipital region. There are two forms of colour agnosia. Firstly a difficulty in identifying colours in daily living. Matching, selecting lighter or deeper shades, or even sorting colours proves extremely difficult or impossible, yet no colour sense disorder is apparent. Tests such as the Ishihara (used to select pilots during wartime) show colour vision is normal. In the other form, colour naming is the problem. The usual tests for colour blindness prove normal and yet the person is unable to name colours or to recognise the name when it is supplied.

The first type of colour disorder is probably related to right hemisphere damage and the latter more related to aphasia. Usually there are other symptoms and signs which help to provide a better picture of the individual problem.

Taste and smell.　　These are not of great importance for the attention of researchers, though they are of importance to the individual. Regarding the elderly it should be remembered that taste and smell are closely linked. Sensory acuity does change with age, and men are more likely to lose acuity of the sense of smell than women. Older people often complain that food does not taste as good as it used to, or that something tastes poisonous. This is due to the changes in the sense of smell which do, for most people, make a meal more appetising. Awareness of these changes can help carers to understand some of the complaints.

Astereognosis

This condition is also called tactile agnosia. Here the patient is unable to recognise objects by touch alone. It is often hard to distinguish this from sensory weakness of the hand, probably more intense with age accompanied by arthritis, and other related disorders. Shape discrimination is probably the most relevant aspect of tactile disorder, and is usually related to right hemisphere lesions. Practically, astereognosis poses added problems for the old and frail. Finding keys in the dark, searching for money in a handbag, all anxiety-provoking or potentially embarrassing situations.

Home helps and other visitors could encourage their clients to find safe and easier ways to identify important objects that they cannot recognise by feel alone. As shape appears to be the main defect, and texture and roughness could well be preserved, something rough could be attached to the key to aid recognition, and weight might be useful with regard to money in a purse.

Unilateral visual inattention

This is an important and far from uncommon state frequently found with stroke patients — though not exclusively so. There are a variety of types and of terminologies for conditions which are essentially disturbances of body image or awareness. *Anosognosia* is a denial of disease and a rejection of body parts that are affected. A paralysed arm will be ignored or even said to belong to someone else. The patient may not even dress that side of the body. All sensory input on the affected side will be ignored — talking to the person on the side that is neglected will elicit no response whatsoever, even food on a plate will be eaten only from one half of the plate, and written words will only be read on the accepted side. Usually attention is directed to the same side as the lesion, and it is the other side of the body that is neglected. The right parietal lobe is the area most commonly affected; hemiparesis is usually, but not always, associated. It also occurs with frontal damage and also with some subcortical lesions. The acute form can become minimal if the patient is making a reasonable recovery, but some signs will persist, though they might become hard to identify.

Autotopagnosia. This is another term for impaired recognition of body parts. *Finger agnosia* is a particular form of this and can easily be tested. The latter forms one of the classical signs denoting Gerstmann's syndrome. The others are agraphia, aculculia and right–left disorientation.

Though discussion ranges wide and long over the real existence of such a syndrome, in practice the presence of at least three of these problems proves very suggestive of a lesion in the left parietal lobe.

Body image disturbance is associated with the parietal lobes; usually the right hemisphere is involved.

Other factors

Areas such as the frontal lobes and subcortical regions play major roles in explanations of unusual behaviour. The slowness, apathy and apparent forgetfulness of a person with a subcortical lesion or disease process (see Chapter 4) can be overlooked and misinterpreted so that the true cause is missed. This is probably due to the word 'dementia' being included in the term, and could provoke a response similar to 'Oh, so, nothing can be done.'

Because these patients respond so slowly it is assumed that they are intellectually, globally deteriorating. The presence of a dysarthria is mistaken for an aphasia, and the absence of any true aphasia or agnosia and apraxia remains unnoticed. Although slowed down, or dilapidated intellectually, patients with subcortical states remain intellectually able until very late in their particular illness. If a person is treated as though he or she has deteriorated, anxiety and depression will be reinforced. Impatient responses or reactions will also affect motivation. Such clients will frequently say 'I don't know' when asked questions. This is often a defence against impatient handling and an expression of feelings of worthlessness. Such patients require support, encouragement, time and a higher level of expectation.

The effects of damage in the frontal areas of the brain are remarkable enough to be referred to as the *frontal lobe syndrome*. Personality changes are marked and, even with the very young, can cause the person to behave in a most unsociable and unacceptable manner.

Impulsivity, outspokenness, poor judgement, mood swings, garrulousness, an inability to understand abstract ideas and inappropriate laughter or weeping are all possible, obviously varying in presence and degree of severity from individual to individual. Abilities are also affected. The person may perseverate, either verbally or with movements. Sequencing and order are impaired; so is logical thought, planning and problem-solving. A common problem is associated with perseveration — an inability to shift set. This results in the person being unable to sort things into different categories or to change from one programme or line of thought to another.

In the mildest states of frontal damage the person is long-winded, rather impulsive and variable in mood, but individual variations must be remembered.

The elderly

As this book is concerned with older people the relevance of neuropsychology to this age group must be considered. In many instances the clients in care are frail and ill, and often standard test procedures are not suitable or desirable. However, it must be stressed that a proper investigation is vital in each case in order to provide logical and sensible grounds for treatment or management programmes. The actual process of investigation will be discussed in Chapter 3, but it is important to recognise the need to obtain as much relevant information about a person as it is possible to do. While there are many who will resent, reject or be unable to respond to formal testing, and therefore more gentle measures are required, not all elderly people are frail and incapable of coping with more formal examinations. The majority of older people are fit, independent and well, and can respond to appropriate investigations. Older people who attend general medical clinics or neurological units are frequently very capable people who, if treated respectfully and allowed to retain their dignity, will be able to cope with the investigations as well as any other age group.

In our eagerness to protect a group from exploitation and embarrassment it remains as important to avoid over-protectiveness and patronisation as it is to put an elderly person under undue stress and unnecessary threat. It is not unusual to discover that the client aged 90 years is more intellectually capable than the examiner!

ALTERNATIVE EXPLANATIONS OF OBSERVED BEHAVIOUR

In this chapter the aim is to suggest more careful assessment of problems. An assessment should not only look at skills, daily living abilities and patterns of behaviour, levels of cognitive and behavioural functioning, environmental and social backgrounds, and interests, but also assist diagnosis and the identification of brain function abilities and impairments. Without such an overall picture mistakes will be made, misinterpretations will occur and improper programme goals will be set. Some of the commonest errors are in misinterpreting behaviour which may well be related to some form of neuropsychological deficit.

17

Table 1.2: Examples of behaviours and possible alternative explanations

Observed behaviours	Alternative explanations to be investigated
Walking into things.	Visual problems. Weakness due to stroke. Alcoholism, tumour, head injury, anosognosia, autotopagnosia.
Drops things, lacks dexterity.	Parkinson's disease, peripheral weakness, apraxia, stroke.
Inappropriate laughing or crying.	Probably frontal lesion.
Gets into someone else's bed, complains of assault.	Probably anosognosia due to stroke, tumour or head injury.
Very slow, little response.	Depression, subcortical state, e.g. Parkinson's disease.
Eats very little.	May be normal habit. Anorexia. Peripheral field problem. Anosognosia.
Will not dress.	Dressing apraxia, agnosia, anosognosia.
Does not recognise faces or objects.	Probably a visual agnosia and/or prosopagnosia.
Sings beautifully, but does not talk.	Melody and music in other hemisphere. Patient is probably aphasic.
Says nothing, or uses nonsense words.	Probably aphasic.
Forgets to pass on a message.	Probably suffering from benign forgetfulness, just like anyone else!

Some of the more common 'soft' signs have been outlined above. The behaviours listed on Table 1.1 can now be re-examined, and some alternative explanations offered.

Walking into things usually implies some form of visual disturbance. There is a very long list of possibilities to be considered. Some of them are obvious — blindness, delirium, limb weakness. Others are not so well known. Strokes, tumours and head injuries can produce body image disturbances such as anosognosia. Here if the object is on the neglected side of the body obviously the patient will not be aware of it. The rare Balint's syndrome — where the patient has a fixation of gaze, an optic ataxia and impaired visual attention — could easily account for clumsiness, tripping and other errors related to not seeing things properly.

Normal gaze is possible until the patient's eyes fix on something; once this happens he or she cannot voluntarily shift that gaze — another kind of apraxia. The optic ataxia causes errors when the person tries to grasp the object on which fixation has occurred — so a cup is spilt or a plate knocked over. Equally the eyes will not account for other objects in the periphery of the object which has caught the gaze. Even if several pencils are lined up together only the one the gaze has settled upon will have any meaning. It is impossible to count the correct number or to distinguish one from another.

Dexterity deficits are rarely pure clumsiness. Tremors, shakes, weaknesses and stiffnesses should be noted, and the possibility of a transient ischaemic attack (TIA) considered. Progressive supranuclear palsy, with its stiffnesses and lack of downward gaze, will make walking, eating and reading or writing a considerable problem, even an impossibility, for the patient. A parkinsonian tremor and the slowness of response of this and other subcortical states are good reasons for clumsiness and apparent lack of motivation and co-operation.

Errors in understanding language difficulties are widespread. Few people appreciate that — though language is, essentially, the concern of the dominant (usually left) hemisphere — music, melody, rhythm, and tempo are usually sited in the right temporal area. As a result of this the 'singer' with aphasia for speech has often been regarded as a malingerer. Sadly a number of famous singers and composers — Ravel for instance — have suffered the tragic fate of developing the opposite disability, an amusia — an impairment in musical appreciation where speech is preserved and music lost. Once again the effects vary; some can hear music in their heads but cannot write, play or sing it; others hear a cacophonous row rather than harmonious melody. As disability can affect the daily work or pleasures of ordinary people it can also affect creative and inventive minds who will suffer from loss just as much as anyone else unless suitable support is offered and further research with rehabilitation in focus is encouraged.

It is advisable, but not always possible, to call on the help of a neuropsychologist, speech therapist or occupational therapist in order to examine problems carefully. Outside neurology few medical specialties are conversant with neuropsychology, and as a result these investigations are frequently overlooked. It is vital to the patient that his or her observed behaviour is understood and related to rehabilitation or management. Simple screening tests are possible, and some knowledge of possible neuropsychological explanations is preferable to total ignorance. Common sense and basic knowledge are reasonable tools. Staff can examine the situation for themselves by making careful enquiries, observations of behaviour and by making careful records. Even so, more training programmes are required.

Regular discussion and consideration of the questionable behaviours and their possible causes would be the proper sequel to an observations period. During this time all retained abilities would be recorded — no matter how basic. A good starting point is to ask 'Does the patient breathe?' The question is a surprise, and at first amusing, but it prompts recall of quite basic positive examples of abilities and simple skills, as well as positive aspects of the individual's personality. The great rush to set targets based on faulty information must be discouraged. In most cases a delay, during which all the person receives is tender loving concern, will do more to assist rehabilitation and provide a better opportunity to assess retained and disabled function than an impressive-looking, but worthless, set of goals.

CASE 1, EXAMPLE

The nurses on a geriatric ward were deeply distressed when Mr Brown and his relatives threatened court action. They claimed that he had been assaulted by one of the night staff. This was denied, and both relatives and staff anxiously sought clarification of the incident.

Mr Brown had suffered a severe stroke which had paralysed his left side. Ten days after the event he was still extremely impaired intellectually and unable to do much for himself. When further investigations were instigated it soon became apparent that he had an agnosognosia and completely ignored his left side. He did not respond to sensory stimuli of any nature presented on his left side. He insisted that his left hand did not belong to him.

The most likely explanation for the reported incident was that during the night the part of his body which he recognised as his own came in contact with the hand he claimed belonged to somebody else. When this possibility was demonstrated to the relatives and staff they were surprised by the existence of such a state, and convinced that this must explain the situation. Although the staff were trained to an excellent standard they had failed to place any relevance to diagnosis on the neglect of one side, and although some of them had noticed that Mr Brown failed to respond to stimuli to that side no record was made of it. If training had included basic neuropsychological signs this would not have happened.

CASE 2, EXAMPLE

Mrs Black was causing concern amongst the residential home care staff. Since her admission to the home some twelve months previously she had begun to deteriorate gradually. Now she appeared unmotivated, unco-operative and very clumsy. She was so messy at mealtimes that they found it easier to feed her themselves. Mornings and evenings were made more demanding for staff as they had to dress and wash her, or she would take hours to complete the tasks on her own.

When observations at different times of the day were taken it was noted that:

1. When left to cope alone Mrs Black did not seem to be clumsy all the time, e.g. she picked up a magazine and turned the pages without any problem, and when a cup of tea was placed beside her she drank it in a normal way.
2. At mealtimes staff would feed her without allowing her to try. Problems intensified when staff said 'Open your mouth, Mrs Brown' or told her to pick something up.
3. When dressing or undressing, the supervising staff member usually completed the task. Invariably requests to 'lift your arm' or 'put your foot in here' met with chaos.

The implications of an apraxia were explained to the staff and *all* staff members were encouraged to avoid directing Mrs Black's attention on to a task. Distracting her attention was stressed. Considerable improvement in self-care was noted. It required a careful step-by-step programme in order to fade out some of the effects of institutionalisation and expectation of dependency, but when staff and client appreciated that it was within Mrs Black's ability to perform movements naturally and automatically she was given much more opportunity and encouragement to care for herself.

REFERENCES

Albert, M. (1981) Geriatric neuropsychology. *Journal of Consulting and Clinical Psychology,* *49*(6), 835–50

Benson, F. (1979) *Aphasia, agraphia, alexia.* Churchill Livingstone, New York

Hecaen, H. and Albert, M.L. (1978) *Human neuropsychology.* John Wiley, New York

Holden, U.P. and Woods, R.T. (1988) *Reality orientation,* 2nd edn. Churchill Livingstone, Edinburgh and New York

Miller, E. (1984) *Recovery and management of neuropsychological impairments.* John Wiley, Chichester and New York

Walsh, K. (1987) *Neuropsychology.* Churchill Livingstone, Edinburgh and New York

2

Realistic Assessment

Una Holden

METHODS IN COMMON PRACTICE

Over the years elderly people have been presented with tests of
various forms which have rarely been of any relevance to their
problems, appropriate to their abilities or capable of reflecting
their interests or needs. They have suffered from the popular
myth which accepts that intellectual deterioration is the natural
accompaniment of increasing age. Intelligence test constructors
obviously supported such a view and ignored variables such as
the fact that a totally different cultural society was in operation
50 or more years ago. People grew up with different health,
nutritional, educational and environmental systems and opportunities. Such tests made direct comparisons between older and
younger age groups with a patronising extra points allowance
for age. By failing to recognise the variables the test constructors provided tools which reinforced the myth which, despite
contrary findings from research programmes, is proving hard to
eradicate. Currently test batteries are still in use, and the belief
that these batteries will provide valid responses remains a fairly
common one. Battery-based investigations are often used in
large-scale projects which include people in the community as
well as institutions. The Wechsler Adult Intelligence Scale continues to be in vogue, and this or whatever battery is fashionable
in that particular area can be used indiscriminantly regardless of
individual differences or special difficulties. Such an assembly-
line process is unlikely to supply a meaningful picture of a
group, let alone an individual. Some basic errors of this
approach include:

The feelings of the participants are ignored.
The nature of most tests is inappropriate.
The questions employed are irrelevant.
The stress factor is increased.
The participants have little comprehension of the purpose of the tests.
There is a lack of comparison between the individual's past and present performance.
The priorities of the elderly are omitted.
There is no neuropsychological component.

If a client feels threatened by a task, fears that he or she could be shamed by incorrect responses, the concern for preserving some dignity and self-esteem can produce reactions of anger, resentment, embarrassment and even depression. Under such conditions the responses can hardly be seen as valid. Most test material is designed for a younger age group and by younger people. Many questions and situations are totally inappropriate for older people — Woods (1982) points out, for instance, that it is rather rare to find an 87-year-old who wants to find her way through a forest! Equally the abilities required by a driving young executive are hardly likely to be of importance to a retired gentleman in his 90s who is more concerned about keeping his home comfortable and himself healthy than about union activities or government policies. Priorities *do* change, though basic interests may not.

To place unnecessary strain on clients will also result in invalid responses. Particularly in large-scale investigations the clients rarely understand the purpose of the tasks before them. A younger, more assertive person will demand a full explanation, but the older one is more inclined to accept a simple outline, and could well be totally unaware of what is really being asked of him or her. Equally, older people might feel obliged to co-operate because the interviewer is 'so nice and kind'. The response could well be what the older person expects the younger one wants to hear!

Comparison of older with younger age groups is not as important, in most cases, as the comparison between the person's past and present performance. Rarely are there questions or tasks in these batteries or tests which throw any light on this important factor. Information about intellectual ability and skilled performance may be desirable, but how can this be evaluated if there is no investigation into possible deficits in brain function? Neuropsychological changes or influences on abilities should play a paramount role in any assessment. The reasons for changes in function and ability can improve understanding, aid in rehabilitation and indicate retained functions which would be relevant in any goal-setting programme.

While it may be of interest, academically, to know how age affects a person's performance, such information is of little help practically. Batteries are for hens, not for people, and even then they are unnatural! They are impersonal, usually irrelevant, stressful and an invasion of privacy (Holden, 1984). This is not to say that a collection of relevant tests should not be maintained in a department. On the contrary it is of great importance to have such a store, so that there is a choice of procedure to meet the needs of each individual client. In the past few years there have been a number of good reviews of test materials and their relevant merits and uses (Woods, 1982; Birren and Schaie, 1985; Woods and Britton, 1985). Consideration of the more general testing of intellectual level and personality is not appropriate in this context. However, there is common ground with any type of investigation which seeks a baseline of ability on which to build, and which provides a suitable setting and environment in which to carry out any necessary investigations.

Reasons for assessing elderly people

These are probably identical to those for assessing any other age group.

1. Obtaining a baseline assessment of function — both what can and what cannot be done — in order to avoid setting unrealistic goals and expectation.
2. To monitor change.
3. To be able to show positive changes to the client and to have convincing evidence for those who need to know — e.g. other staff, relatives.
4. For selection purposes — to ensure that people of similar levels are in a group programme.
5. Research purposes.

6. For the evaluation of a new approach, treatment programme, service, etc.
7. Assisting diagnosis and prognosis.
8. For legal purposes, e.g. head injury.

Routine assessments on admission to hospital or home are not acceptable for that reason alone, nor are routine administrations of a given test acceptable — an individual's needs are paramount.

When routine testing occurs either invalid results are accepted or a client will respond in a typical manner. The examiner can be told to 'go away'; is ignored or even subjected to an indignant, aggressive outburst. It is quite common to hear a threatened old person say 'I'm sorry I must go and get my mother's tea', or 'I'm afraid I haven't got my glasses with me' or even as a last resort 'Please ask my daughter that, she will know the answer'. The elderly are basically very polite; they often do not wish to offend and find the avoidance excuses the best way to escape. It is also possible that, as they do not quite understand why they are being asked these questions, a daughter *would* be more helpful to the enquiry. It is hardly surprising that door-to-door salesmen manage to trick the old so easily. As most test responses are so obviously dubious it is hard to accept that many 'findings' based on such investigations are of any value.

The myth regarding the loss of intellectual ability with increasing age has been unmasked by researchers such as Schaie and his colleagues (1968, 1974). Many workers are showing that intelligent young people will probably become intelligent older ones as a vast number of older superpersons have been overlooked in the concern about what to do for the deteriorating mentally infirm elderly. It is important to appreciate that as there are people more intelligent than ourselves quite a number of those include older people in care, and this group will find it very exasperating to be treated as intellectually inferior to their supporters.

Preparation for assessment

Before any investigations are initiated consideration should be given as to the aims of that investigation and also to the circumstances in which it will be carried out. Where is it going to be? What was the stated problem to be investigated and what is known already about that person?

The first step should always be to obtain information about the person's background and history. A team with a social worker will be at an advantage, but there are other questions that other members of a team would require answering. Difficulties arise when the client is very confused or unwell. There may be no surviving relative to answer questions, long-time friends may have died or moved away, the neighbours may have little to tell. The social worker can pick up some clues from the home — photographs, the house and possessions, various souvenirs — all of these can provide some help in the search for previous levels of life experience. Usually relatives or the person himself or herself can fill in useful details. Neighbours will know about routines, likes and some of the person's habits and interests. Even a forgetful rather vague old person can provide many indications of previous standards. Previous occupations, education, travel, skills and interests, the occupations of other relatives, can all aid in building up a picture of the whole person.

To be able to evaluate the significance of any responses to test procedures it is important to know if there is a noticeable discrepancy between present functioning and that which was in operation before the person became ill. It is difficult, it can never be clear-cut — for instance a person may have had the potential ability to lead a most successful life and yet never had the opportunity. With those who are highly intelligent it is often hard to detect a genuine loss; equally with those who were not so intelligent it is easy to assume a loss.

Without some baseline indication of ability it is extremely hard to evaluate performance on tasks, or to set realistic and appropriate goals. *If* the person is capable of completing a formal test, when a good rapport has been established, a test such as the National Adult Reading Test (NART) developed by Nelson (1982) could prove useful. Any difficulty with language would make it useless, but generally it does give a good indication of the person's previous educational level. If the words are reprinted in larger type it becomes more of an eyesight test than a threatening vocabulary or reading test! The more able can also respond with interest to a gently introduced Block Design test or to Raven's Coloured Matrices. With most older, infirm people the latter two should be avoided.

Most early investigators arrived at an interview with a client carrying a case-full of test materials. Today it is more acceptable simply to sit down and talk. Establishing a good rapport is vital. Some social contact is important to the person, who also needs a rebuilding of confidence. Hospital or a home may be very nice, but it is not the *real* home and can disorient or threaten the person. A client requires a feeling of ease and reasonable control over a situation before he or she can respond to enquiries which could be interpreted as an invasion of privacy. An experienced and understanding clinician or therapist will take time to allow the person to maintain dignity and to be able to respond without embarrassment or nervousness. All investigators should be aware of this. Before goals can be set it is important to identify the strengths and weaknesses. Activities of daily living (ADL) and the intellectual levels are important once the medical situation has been checked. Information from all branches of a team is necessary (Wattis and Church, 1986), before conclusions can be reached. This information is relevant to the process of rehabilitation, retraining and treatment. However, although books and training in all professions concerned provide information on good standards of practice, brain function is rarely included. It is unusual for staff to consider the implications of behaviour and ability in this light. To omit neuropsychological implications can lead to setting impossible and even meaningless goals.

NEUROPSYCHOLOGICAL INVESTIGATIONS

Neuropsychological batteries

Marilyn Albert's classical article on geriatric neuropsychology (1981) provides a good overview of the problems, and stresses the need to understand the neuropsychological profile of each disorder. Amongst the batteries the most widely known are:

The Halstead–Reitan.
The Golden–Nebraska.
Wechsler's Adult Intelligence Scale.
Luria's Neuropsychological Investigation (Christensen, 1975).

There are a number of other batteries which have a limited popularity and a variety of useful tests for specific abilities, e.g. the Boston Diagnostic Aphasia Examination (Goodglass and Kaplan, 1972) and the Rivermead Behavioural Memory Test (Wilson and Moffat, 1984).

There is not a great deal to be said about test batteries that has not been covered in the early pages of this chapter. With regard to the use of the Wechsler Adult Intelligence Scale (WAIS) as a neuropsychological tool to investigate the difficulties of any age group articles have been written in protest for so many years that there are not enough pages in this chapter to include them (e.g. Albert, 1981; Satz and Fletcher, 1981; Woods and Britton, 1985).

The merits or demerits of the Halstead–Reitan Battery have also led to much discussion, but its length, types of subtest and the practice of using technicians to present it make it inappropriate for elderly clients anyway. It would be easy to become embroiled in the Golden–Nebraska controversy (Spiers, 1981), but as this battery is also inappropriate discussion of its use of the Luria material will be avoided.

Of all the investigations mentioned above, probably only Anne-Lise Christensen's version of Luria's work is of relevance. Even here a long, complicated series of tests can prove a problem, but then Luria himself would not have used the whole investigation, only wishing to find that which would tell him what he wanted to know. A careful selection of items from the different sections proves a valuable aid to assessing most of the old people who are capable of coping with a set test situation. It is even possible to use many of the items at a bedside. A recent study by Blackburn and Tyrer (1985) successfully distinguished between Alzheimer's disease, Korsakov's and control subjects. They used a shortened version of the Luria which included tasks from all sections. It is interesting to note that most of the tests were attempted by the subjects.

It is Luria's belief in the need to observe and to use common sense which should be the guide for assessing the majority of elderly people. The most important question in examining for brain function and ability is *can the person do this or can he or she not do it?* It is not a question of how does this person of over 70 years compare in performance with a 20-year-old. It is the business of a neuropsychologist to have a collection of tests rather than a battery, and to select those that are relevant to further investigate the findings of a screening procedure. Many elderly persons will respond well to more demanding situations if the purpose is sensitively and properly explained.

Major problems arise when working with the large number of fragile, unresponsive or very confused clients. It is here that the clinician's imagination, observational abilities and experience become important. Where the investigator lacks an appreciation of neuropsychological factors, and has limited knowledge of the implications of particular behaviours, he or she is more prone to feelings of frustration, annoyance and impatience. Under these circumstances the client can be reported as being 'untestable, obviously very deteriorated'. What *is* obvious here is the lack of experience and ability of the investigator.

Practical or basic neuropsychological investigations

In Chapter 1 definitions were provided for most of the terms used to describe the 'soft signs' of neuropsychology, as they are called.

Ideally, for a thorough investigation, the help of a neuropsychologist should be sought. As many units do not have a neuropsychologist on whom to call, staff should have sufficient knowledge of some of the basic problems. These can be observed or indicated by simple screening methods and should be used by all those working with older people exhibiting disorders of ability and behaviour. Common sense remains the most important and least-employed approach of all, and with some additional knowledge and skill most staff can find an explanation for their 'instinctive' feelings about their clients. Not all situations call for a comprehensive and in-depth assessment.

If an individual is very lucid, fluent and obviously capable of managing his or her own affairs and life, it is highly unlikely that aid, other than that of a medical nature, will be required. A person who reads the newspaper, directional signs, forms and letters with ease will not require lengthy investigations of reading ability. Also, if the person has forgotten to bring along the necessary reading glasses it is rather stupid to conclude that there is a dyslexia problem!

Though it might appear obvious it is surprising how often lack of teeth, hearing aids or glasses lead the observer to remarkable conclusions! Laterality is another obvious but forgotten clue. With older people in particular it is advisable to establish early in the investigation if they are right- or left-handed. Many were forced to use their right hand in school instead of the preferred left hand — usually because it was regarded as more socially acceptable. To omit to check this can lead to misinterpretation and misunderstanding of behaviour and responses. Diagnostic difficulties can be caused by an apparently right-handed person who shows no evidence of language deficits, despite right-sided paralysis. The real impairments with space and perception are overlooked, so a vascular accident in a person who may be right hemisphere dominant can be missed.

The examination setting should give consideration to the following:

The atmosphere during investigations should be as relaxed as possible.

The tasks should be geared to the individual.

The interests, social skills, experience and standards learned from initial enquiries should be used as far as possible.

The situation should be friendly, warm and encouraging without being intrusive.

The aim should be to encourage the person to succeed as well as possible.

The interview should be short. A little at a time is better than too much at once.

It is better to simply talk at the first meeting than to push too hard and lose the person's confidence.

The investigation should be geared to finding the person's *retained* abilities as well as the impaired or lost ones.

Different neuropsychologists lay emphasis on different areas of function to be examined. They also work in different ways. Albert (1981), for instance emphasises: attention, language, memory, visuo-spatial ability, cognitive flexibility and abstraction. Others either have a list of areas that they seek out during the investigation, or develop a mental picture of the areas so that when they have completed their investigation they are able to link the responses together into a meaningful whole. Most staff, untrained in the field of neuropsychology, are recommended to use a list containing the major headings and including simple tests for screening purposes. It is wise to remember that one failure does not imply genuine damage or an impairment,

Table 2.1: Areas of investigation

Previous history and basic ability.
Laterality.
Orientation.
Acquired knowledge.
Aphasia: dysarthria; fluent or non-fluent speech difficulties; comprehension; agraphia; acalculia; alexia.
Apraxia: ideomotor; ideational; constructional; dressing.
Agnosia: visual or object; spatial; anosognosia, prosopagnosia; possibly simultanagnosia, though further investigations by trained staff are advisable if this is suspected.
Memory: short-term; long-term; delayed; visual and spatial.
Frontal signs: garrulousness; personality change; poor logic and sequencing; poor judgement and planning; perseveration; inability to think in the abstract; inability to change set — the 'stuck needle' syndrome.
Subcortical signs: slowness; slow, dysarthric or minimal speech; apathy or aggression; forgetfulness — forgetting to remember; acquired knowledge difficulties; no aphasia, apraxia or agnosia.

but suggests further investigations. Most people have particular strengths and weaknesses in ability. For example there are those who cannot tell left from right, and yet they do not necessarily have an impairment of brain function which requires treatment — a little retraining perhaps! Some people find their way by road signs and numbers, others look for buildings and landmarks. Everyone is different, so single errors may be of no significance whatsoever. When tasks related to a specific ability are regularly failed, the evidence is more convincing. However, even minor errors are worth recording as they serve as a means of checking on a possibly developing problem — or may even be a sign of recovery.

The list of areas to investigate could include those listed in Table 2.1. Attention, and the length of time a person can maintain concentration are other important factors.

In many cases it will not be necessary to test for all these signs or disorders. Observation and common sense will provide many of the answers.

Initial meeting

The nature of the initial contact depends on the circumstances and the client's degree of disorder. If the person is at home and fairly independent it is possible to talk about the problems, to elicit a little about the person's history and perhaps include some relevant tests. At the same time the reason for the meeting can be explained, and reassurance given that it is the person's strengths that are most important as it is those abilities which will be used to help the weaker ones improve, or find alternative ways to manage. Generally the client is in hospital or a residential home. Here it is important to establish a good social relationship. Introductions and explanations — quite simple ones — are required.

The person should be encouraged to talk about him/herself and about both the past and the present.

One of the most important things about medical training is that it teaches its future doctors to use their eyes and ears. It is unfortunate that other professions do not receive similar instructions. It is also sad that this important feature of an examination is so easily forgotten.

All care workers have the opportunity to observe. Eyes and ears provide invaluable information without a single question being asked.

Listen

It is easy to hear what is being said, providing hearing is not defective. The content of the conversation is important, but also how it is said, what response is made, how words are formed and used, what sentences are like, and how well the person expresses ideas, are all of vital importance.

Aphasia — speech
Careful attention will distinguish a dysarthria from a dysphasia.

Dysarthria. Here the sentence structure and words will be correct or near-normal, but the production of sound is guttural, thick, slurred and very low-pitched or indistinct.

Anomia. This can be picked up by the roundabout way a person tries to get across the meaning of a word instead of using the proper word, e.g. 'Well, that longish thing used to write with, it has ink in it' could be used instead of 'pen'. This is a word-finding difficulty.

Festination. Refers to the little staccato noises made by a patient with Parkinson's disease as he or she begins to speak. It sounds almost like a stutter of 'ehs', but once started the 'eh-eh-eh-ehs' cease. The person may also speak very, very quietly and be almost inaudible.

Expressive or non-fluent aphasia. This is usually easy to detect. The person may not be able to speak at all, say only 'yes' and 'no', or use particular words or phrases repeatedly with different emphases as though really expressing him/herself. 'I don't know what to say', 'Five, five, five' are just examples of many variations. Social phrases are often preserved and lead others to believe all is well. Rhythm and prosody can also be preserved and can be employed to give meaning, or apparent meaning, to the few words actually spoken. When speech is so limited the difficulty is obvious. However, sometimes it is not so obvious and careful listening is needed to detect an anomia, wrong beginnings to a word, mixed-up parts of a word or missing parts of a sentence (see Chapter 5).

Fluent or receptive dysphasia. This may be missed or misunderstood. The lack of response or strange response of a patient can be interpreted in many ways. By listening to responses to questions the inappropriateness becomes more obvious. The attempts to communicate are also helpful. Words and apparent sentences will be used, but they can be meaningless or obscure. Frequently the person becomes upset or irritated as the listener does not understand what is being said. Often the client is unaware of the problem. The help of a speech therapist at this point is highly desirable, as the problem is not a straightforward one.

Aphasia — alexia (reading)

In a sociable manner it is acceptable to encourage a person to read from the newspaper or a magazine — ensuring that if glasses are required they are in use. Listen to see if the patients read correctly — it will also be necessary to watch. Do they miss words, lines, or part of the page? If there are letters or cards, do they recognise the writing of close relatives and friends? Do they read the signs on the ward without any problem? By conducting this enquiry in a natural manner the person should be able to respond naturally too. 'Can you find your way around the ward yet? Let's see, can you see the sign for the bathroom from here? It looks a bit small to me, can you really read it?'

Using newspapers or journals in a similarly chatty manner will soon elicit evidence of an ability, or lack of an ability, to read, even if it is only the large letters. It is important to ascertain if the patient understands what has been read, so some discussion on the topic will be helpful. The objects of a personal nature around the bedside or table can prove useful. A box of talcum powder, for instance, provides the opportunity to say 'My mother used to like that powder, what's it called? Oh yes — can you see — it has the name there?' By encouraging the person to read the writing on the box — or whatever — it is possible to get further insight not only into reading ability, but also recognition and possibly memory.

Although this discussion on how to listen and what to hear is concentrating on one possibility at a time, factors other than language skills can be screened. During conversation it is possible to notice perseverations other than the aphasic repetition of one word or phrase.

Perseveration. This implies that, although a person speaks normally most of the time, every so often a phrase or thought is repeated again and again (see Chapter 1). This repetition is more likely to occur when the person is not being given attention and is sitting alone, but it does happen during conversation too, and should be noted. This is common to clients with some degree of frontal damage.

Mutism. Mutism — no speech at all — should also be noted, though this can be due to a variety of reasons including subcortical states and psychiatric ones. Slowness of speech and of response is another noteworthy finding, and could be due to Parkinson's disease or other subcortical states.

Confabulation. This is yet another problem that can be highlighted during a conversation. Korsakov's patients often make up convincing responses to questions which usually concern the past, though it can be about the present too. The content of the response is often mistaken for delusions. One lady, when asked where she was (in hospital), replied that the year was 1925 and she was at a picnic, and that the lady sitting across from her was her sister. She was probably recalling a real picnic with her family at about that time ... who can tell?

Psychiatric disturbances such as hallucinations, delusions and paranoid ideas can also be picked up by listening to a person's flow of conversation. However, it is wise to ascertain if what appears paranoid has not really happened! There is always an elderly apparently confused person who talks about noises and giggling outside her window, and people trying to frighten her, who could well have been persecuted by thoughtless, naughty children, or even a more serious intruder. There is also the 'deluded' lady who really *did* have tea with the Queen last weekend!

If nothing else, a good listener can learn a great deal about an individual's background, personal needs, experiences and habits, as well as about the environment and normal day-to-day living patterns. All of this can prove vital to successful goal-setting — or simple common-sense ways to help the person regain at least some independence.

Agnosias

By standing on one side of a person (usually the left side) and talking, it is easily established whether or not the person is ignoring or reacting normally to that side. If there is no response try touching or movement. Move to a central position in front of the person and try again. If response only comes from one side to more or less the middle of the person's nose it is very possible that there is an *anosognosia* or one-sided neglect present.

If a person fails to recognise or respond even to familiar people until they speak then it is possible that there is a disturbance of facial recognition (*prosopagnosia*). This problem is not uncommon, and can be the only difficulty that a family will complain about. It can include the client's own face — not recognising a reflection in the mirror. One couple had great difficulties, as every time the husband saw his own reflection he accused his 75-year-old wife of having a lover. Apart from that he was no problem. He was unable to recognise anyone else's face in a mirror either. Many women fail suddenly to recognise their husbands. Though there may well be a useful avoidance element present, this is hard to prove! One 70-year-old insisted that her husband was her father. Though she was able to recognise the difference with photographs (usually the most vulnerable to facial recognition problems) she insisted that the living man was not her husband. In some cases there might be an element of rejection or wishful thinking, and some psychopathology might be present; usually there is an organic basis. One lady asked for advice about the strange man who insisted that as her husband he had a right to go to bed with her. She was deeply concerned about the moral issue but added 'he is gorgeous, you know'. Needless to say the therapist advised her to enjoy the relationship! Face recognition problems can be elicited not only by failure to recognise family and friends but also by an inability to recognise famous faces in magazines or newspapers. So, yet again, a conversation can prove useful.

Watching

Watching how a person behaves, reacts and moves can provide many clues to the nature of the person's problem.

Hands. Look for tremor, hand-wringing, tapping and impaired gesture.

Apraxias

Gesture may be an attempt to communicate, and if the person has language difficulties this may be the only form of expression possible. Gesture is also important in establishing the presence of an apraxia. By asking a person to pretend to wave, to brush his/her hair or clean his/her teeth an inability to perform an action on request can be highlighted. Watch to see if the person performs the action without prompting.

Notice what happens when a person is given a plate of food and the staff member says 'Pick up your knife and fork and eat your lunch'. Do the hands get mixed up and awkward, is the cutlery item dropped, held awkwardly and are hand movements so clumsy that the staff member has to help? If the food is presented without instruction, and merely accompanied by a comment such as 'Lunch looks nice today', will the person cope normally? This impairment of simple gesture could be an *ideo-motor apraxia*.

Ideational apraxia. This is shown by mistakes made in the series of actions required to complete a task. The classical test of this is to ask the client to strike a match and light a candle. Another possibility is to ask 'Please would you take some of the matches out of this box and put them in this empty one?', or

'Here is some money, would you count out six pennies and put them in this purse, please?'

In each case a person with ideational apraxia would mix up the sequences and be unable to perform the task in the order necessary. The matches would probably be on the floor and the pennies scattered. In each case — ideational and ideomotor — the patient will be able to perform actions automatically, or when attention is not drawn to the detail.

Constructional apraxia. This condition is more common than realised. The lady who was a productive knitter suddenly has problems with a pattern. The cook gets the ingredients wrong — too much, too little or none at all. The car mechanic cannot put the engine back together. Sometimes this condition can be observed, but it is often not easy to establish by observation. Even so it is important to avoid jumping to conclusions on the basis of one sort of failure. To provide more evidence try jigsaws, mosaics, the Block Design test from the Wechsler or some drawings. Can the person draw a square, cube or box, a star or a clock face saying ten to five? Many people have difficulty with drawing stars and other shapes, so allowance does need to be made for this. If the clinician draws a model to copy this can help, particularly with those who have a dominant hemisphere lesion, but it makes things much worse for those with damage on the non-dominant side as it means that they have more spatial organisation to cope with than they can manage. Similarly with the Block Design — the pictures of patterns add to the confusion if right-sided damage is present. Match or cocktail sticks can be used to form star or other shapes.

The clock drawing is useful in demonstrating left-sided neglect. Half of the drawing will be omitted, or the numbers will be squashed into one side only. Using an actual clock shape with removable parts can also be valuable in showing neglect or constructional problems.

Dressing apraxia. This is probably one of the most-overlooked problems on a ward. Here misunderstanding is the rule, and the patient is believed to be unco-operative or unmotivated. Very often a person has great difficulty in relating the clothes to his or her own person. There could also be a problem in sorting out which are clothes and which is the surface on which they are laid — a figure–ground disturbance. Admittedly the person could be being difficult, but the chances are high that this is related to brain function impairment of some kind. It might even be due to subcortical slowness. If there are dressing delays and difficulties it is advisable to assume that this is related to a specific problem.

Agnosias

Is it necessary for a person to pick up an object, examine it tactilely, put it to the nose to smell it, or put it in the mouth to taste it before working out what it is? Does the person look about in puzzlement for an object and not be able to visually distinguish it until it is actually in his or her hands, or can be touched? This would suggest an inability to visually recognise an object. It is probably reflecting a visual agnosia, but there are other disturbances that may be involved — e.g. a Balint's syndrome. Medical and neurological advice should be sought.

Frontal signs

Watch for repetitive movements and gestures. Simple hand movement sequences as suggested by Luria (Christensen, 1975) can show sequence difficulties: 'When I knock once, you knock twice. When I knock twice you knock once.' Simultaneously having one fist clenched and the other hand open, and then alternating the open and closed hands rhythmically, will demonstrate a possible difficulty when the person has both hands open or both fists clenched.

Touching each finger with the thumb, and at the same time counting 'One, two, three, four' fairly quickly, one hand at a time, is another hand sequencing test. Or with both hands moving at once the patient is asked to say and move hands to match 'Fist, Edge (edge of hands) Palm'. With each of these the sequence should first be demonstrated.

An inability to understand how to put together cartoon pictures so that they make a sensible story can provide yet another use for a newspaper. It also shows an inability to deal with sequences and logic.

Tremors and stiffness of hands suggests a medical cause — arthritis or Parkinson's disease for instance — and should be appropriately investigated. It could also suggest the presence of anxiety, as can hand-wringing.

Agraphia. This can also be observed. Can the person write, can he or she hold a pen or pencil properly? If he or she can, does he or she make sense, are there many errors or only a few?

One of the first things to notice is a hemiparesis. If the hand or arm is paralysed the person will obviously have particular problems. It is, though, also worth watching fine movement and noting if the fingers are stiff or clubbed. Once again these are medical problems and should be so treated. Picking and pulling at cloth, objects or even the self can suggest Alzheimer's disease. Slow movements might imply a subcortical state and choreiform ones a Huntington's chorea.

Anosognosia. While listening, left-sided neglect can be suggested if the person fails to respond to stimuli from one side of the body. Further evidence of this can be obtained by watching. Check if the person reads from left to right or only near to the right side of the right-hand page of a journal. Is food left on one side of the plate? Does the person get into bed with someone else because his/her own bed is in the non-perceived world? The person will walk into objects in the way on the neglected side. Occasionally the person will deny the existence of the hand, or even that part of the body, where damage has occurred. He or she will even neglect to dress the neglected side. Sometimes finding that arm in bed will cause a patient to complain of being assaulted, and this will require careful explanations to relations, and much reassurance. Spatial problems can often be observed when a previously capable person is suddenly unable to find the way, or even to read a map. In many cases where the left parietal lobe is damaged a person might not be even capable of finding rooms in his or her own home.

Face

A facial expression can be an aid to diagnosis. A fixed face suggests Parkinson's disease. Staring eyes that cannot look down suggest progressive supranuclear palsy. The same patient will dribble food over clothes and walk with small feeling steps owing to the inability to see downwards properly.

Inappropriate tears and laughter suggest frontal or subcortical conditions. Closed eyes and lack of response over a fair length of time might imply boredom, sleep, a coma, or a wish to be left alone. They could also imply a well-developed and untreated Parkinson's disease. Enquire if recent behaviour was agitated and even aggressive, causing concern to relatives and staff. This evidence of a late stage of the disease is becoming increasingly rare as most cases are identified and treated early, but it does still appear.

Apathy and disinterest are as easy to recognise as elation. All can indicate personality changes, a clue to frontal damage; the first two are more likely to indicate a depression. Smiling depression also occurs.

Twitches, mouthings, and chewing are often closely related to Alzheimer's disease, but can also be drug side-effects, and should be checked medically. Inability to visually scan, too much scanning, fixation of the eyes and visual field deficits are all notable signs of specific conditions, such as Balint's syndrome, and require neurological investigations.

Movements

Watching the way a person *moves* is also of value. Patients may not move at all. Parkinson patients often have grave difficulty in initiating movement, and, once started, can have difficulty in stopping. The tiny shuffling steps, or festination of movement, have already been mentioned.

Those with a subcortical condition may have great difficulty in moving faster than a snail's pace. Hand movements, walking, speech, gesture, any body movements are all markedly slow.

Walking into objects may be due to forgetfulness, or visual problems, but it could also be due to neglect of one side.

Sounds

Hearing may have some impairment, or there may be an auditory agnosia if a person fails to jump at a threatening noise.

Auditory agnosia. This may be related to words, to non-verbal sound or to both. Those with agnosia for speech will complain that everyone is talking 'Double Dutch', those with non-verbal sound problems will not be able to recognise a car horn, a dog barking or any noise for which they cannot see the source.

Memory

This is usually examined by several of the standard tests for screening purposes. More simple measures can be used. Natural questions in conversation are useful: 'What did you have for dinner?', 'Who came to visit you today?' Does the person remember the names of staff, recent national, local or international events? In group therapy memory games, such as Kim's Game, will provide some guide to the person's abilities.

Memory is not only concerned with recent and long-term verbal material. There are many aspects to memory and a few simple tests will not tap them all. The Luria Neuropsychological Investigation (Christensen, 1975) has a valuable section on memory, and many of the subtests can be used with the elderly frail. For instance the person might be asked to remember some words:

house   moon   street   boy   water,

but before being asked to recall them memory is delayed by being required to describe a picture.

Short fables can be used to see how much the person can recall of the content:

The hen and the golden eggs
A man had a hen which laid golden eggs. Wishing to obtain more gold without having to wait for it he killed the hen. But he found nothing inside it, for it was just like any other hen.

Understanding as well as memory can be tested with this — providing the person is willing and capable of co-operating. Another simple task would be to present two sentences:

In the morning the sun rises in the east.
In May the apple trees blossom.

'Please would you repeat the first sentence ... good ... now would you try to remember the second one?' Cards with coloured shapes can be used to tap non-verbal memory. The person is asked to look for ten seconds at a card on which is a large red rectangle, then a blue rectangle is presented. 'Is this the same as the last card?' The next card has on it a red triangle, a blue rectangle and a green circle. After ten seconds the card with a red triangle, green rectangle, and a blue circle is presented and the question repeated. The third card is uncoloured and has a square, a circle, a triangle, a cross and a diamond. After ten seconds the patient is asked either to draw from memory or recall the shapes on the card.

Williams (1973) produced a useful verbal–non-verbal memory test with a delayed recall element in it which is reasonably non-threatening to the not too frail.

These kinds of tests are of little value for investigating memory levels with the very mentally frail. In such cases the material employed in Mental Status Questionnaires is probably sufficient. The CAPE (Pattie and Gilleard, 1979) with its sections on general information, recall of the ABC and counting up to 20, its reading and writing tasks are all that can be asked of severely impaired clients.

Orientation

Mental Status Questionnaires that can be disguised in a conversation make questioning about days, dates, places and persons less threatening. The importance of temporal orientation has been overstressed in examination, and many healthy people of all ages forget the actual day without a ready cue (Brotchie *et al.*, 1985). Those in hospital or care rarely have a good reason to regard one day as being any different from the next. Orientation for place, person, year and season are more important.

Acquired knowledge

This is mainly covered under language, particularly under reading skills and agraphia. The CAPE also provides some basic-level tests. It is easy enough to provide a sentence or some practical calculations, e.g. Please would you write/read:

> The girl has a nice dress.
> Persistence is essential to success.
> If oranges cost 10p/c how much would you have to give the grocer to pay for six oranges?
> If six journals cost 25p/c each how much change would there be from £/$2?

43

Harder problems can be found in the Wechsler, Luria or other intelligence tests. It is worth asking the client to write numbers down from 'dictation', e.g. 46, 267, 9481. Most clients can manage this with ease, others correctly write the first two then once thousands are reached write 900040081, or a similar pattern. This is very suggestive of an Alzheimer's disease, but anxiety or poor education could also be a cause.

Luria offers some relevant tests for acalculia:

$$10 \quad 2 = 20$$
$$10 \quad 2 = 12$$
$$10 \quad 2 = 8$$
$$10 \quad 2 = 5$$

What are the missing arithmetical signs?

$$12 - \quad = 8$$
$$12 + \quad = 19$$

What are the missing numbers?

Frontal lobe involvement

Damage to the frontal lobes can result from head injury, strokes, tumours, dementia-related states and subcortical conditions. With elderly people it is always advisable to check for its presence.

Perseveration.   The old lady who upsets everyone by her constant repetitive shouting of a particular phrase may well have some damage frontally.

Ideas and actions can be repeated too. In most cases it is obvious, but sometimes only drawing and writing tasks can clearly elicit this. While writing a paragraph a word will be repeated again and again. While drawing, the same drawing or part of the drawing will reappear inappropriately elsewhere. When asked to remember a series of words or pictures one of two items will be repeated on several occasions.

The 'stuck-needle' syndrome.   This occurs when a person is asked to respond to a question or to converse normally; then, suddenly, he or she will get stuck with a subject, or even phrase, and will be unable to move from it. No matter what is said the thought cannot be shifted, and the person continues to talk about the subject or repeat the phrase; just like a sticking gramophone needle that has to be moved before the record will continue to play properly. The responses sound like those of a person with a fluent aphasia and can be mistaken for this. Some noise or movement will intervene, and for a time the person responds to the conversation normally once again. In due course the needle sticks again and the repetition commences once more.

Sequencing problems.   A difficulty in ordering things can be tested by some of the subtests of the Luria. Here the client is asked to sort pictures of day-to-day activities into meaningful order. These include pictures of the seasons, the making of a sandwich and the development of a potato plant. Most occupational therapy departments have pictured series of various daily living tasks, and these are ideal for testing for sequencing difficulties.

People with frontal damage have difficulty in dealing with abstract thought. They find it hard to see the implications of sayings such as 'A rolling stone gathers no moss', their explanation of its meaning will remain in the concrete. 'Well, if it keeps rolling the moss will get rubbed off and won't have time to grow'! It is advisable to keep this in mind when trying to explain things to them. Using comparisons will prove more confusing.

Inability to change set is another kind of stuck-needle syndrome. When asked to sort things into groups, e.g. coloured shapes, patients will be able to sort them into one kind of group, but will find it impossible to further sort them into another. Either colour or shape will be chosen, and then a move to the other will prove impossible.

Impaired judgement, reasoning and planning, as well as personality changes, commonly occur where there is some frontal involvement.

Further comments

In most neuropsychological investigations with younger people it is necessary to take great care and time in order to be certain

45

that the results are correctly interpreted. Neuropsychologists have their own selection of test materials and approaches which vary from unit to unit. However, when working with the frail elderly — both physically and mentally — the stress factor is usually much greater and the person's resilience much less. To use well-established procedures as, e.g. Bender apraxia, Boston Aphasia, would not be possible or appropriate. In many cases only screening is possible accompanied by simple procedures, short sessions and a good social atmosphere. The system of talking, watching and listening, as outlined above, is probably the best way to obtain relevant information. It requires the staff member to have a notebook, a list covering areas of function to be checked and a little imagination plus a lot of tactful concern.

On several occasions throughout this chapter mention has been made of newspapers and magazines as aids to conversation. These can form the basis of a simple investigation on screening process (Holden and Woods, 1988). Most hospitals and homes have a selection of journals in the sitting rooms, and so it is natural to use them in a conversational manner. To sit

Table 2.2: Information to be elicited using magazine pages

Dyslexia	Can the person read — even just the large print? Can the person understand what is read?
Prosopagnosia	Is the familiar face recognised?
Simultanagnosia	Can the person appreciate the *whole* picture on a page, or only recognise and describe parts of it?
Colour agnosia	Are the colours recognised? Can they be matched to something around or on the person?
Anosognosia	Where does the person begin to read? Is it, as normal, from left to right, or does reading commence nearer to the right-hand edge of the journal? Are some letters missed off the beginning of the left-hand side of the columns?
Memory	Can the person talk about things, events, etc., related either to the pictures or the information or advertisements on the pages? Can the person recall life events that have just occurred or are about to occur?
Apraxias	Can he or she point to items, pick up the magazine, turn the pages on request or match things in the room to things on the pages?
Comprehension	Does he or she understand what the pictures and articles are about?
Attention	Can the person concentrate for a reasonable period of time on the magazine and on the discussion?
Speech	How clear is the person's speech? Are there any errors, difficulties or communication problems?

with a person examining a magazine or newspaper is seen as a social encounter rather than as a threat. Thumbing through the pages, making comments on the contents and pictures until the right kind of page is found lessens apprehension, and is perceived as a natural thing to do. Ideally the pages that are most useful are those where the left-hand page is a full-page or almost full-page picture or photograph, preferably in colour — usually an advertisement. The right-hand page should be broken up with pictures, drawings, columns of words, large and small print, and, if possible, a picture of a well-known person. In other words a typical magazine layout. This layout makes it possible to screen for a variety of possible problems in a very easy relaxed manner.

Items listed in Table 2.2 may not cover everything, but in a pleasant, short space of time a great deal of information can be gained painlessly. This could form the basis for further investigation of particular possibilities highlighted in the session. It will also serve in gaining the person's confidence and trust, whilst eliminating the threat factor of a structured and formal examination which would be more stressful and possibly embarrassing.

GOAL SETTING

In any rehabilitation programme planning plays a major role. Patients have a variety of problems and it is often hard to ascertain priorities. Frequently goals that are unrealistic are set. Such mistakes guarantee that a person will experience yet more failure, and confidence and self-esteem will receive further blows. One of the errors here is in forgetting that people with damage to brain function are unlikely to return to being as able as they were ten or more years ago. Disability has to be taken into account, but retained ability must also be sought. Goal-setting of a positive nature will be discussed in a later chapter, but here it is important to stress that part of the foundations for good rehabilitation is a good relevant assessment. This must include neuropsychological aspects as well as daily living skills, intelligence, etc.

While it might be obvious that an amputee cannot expect to regain the agility previously taken as a matter of course, it is often not so obvious that certain 'hidden' functions have been severely damaged.

47

Goals can be set which appear reasonable, but because of the lack of understanding of hidden disabilities these goals will never be achieved. Other errors occur in planning unrealistic stages to reach the goals. To use an easy example:

Example: Mrs Jones has difficulty in speaking

Staff have set a goal as: Mrs Jones will speak fluently. This could be unrealistic for many reasons. If Mrs Jones has a dysphasia rather than a sore throat it will be necessary to discover the nature and degree of the problem first. An interim goal of a more appropriate nature might be able to help Mrs Jones to find a useful way to communicate her needs.

With the same lady unrealistic stages proposed could have been:

(a) Every time Mrs Jones makes a noise we will praise her and give her more attention.
(b) After she makes more and more noises we will only give her praise for the use of a word.
(c) We will only give attention and praise when she uses a sentence.

Hopefully no-one would set such stages, but anything is possible! The number of dangers of such staging are legion. The lady in question was not consulted. Reinforcing noise will probably lead to a very disturbed ward and some anxious patients and staff. The chance of the lady ever reaching stage (b) is highly improbable as the poor soul is to be given no retraining on how to make sound, to control it or even how to relate words to objects or anything of meaning to her or to anyone else. The damage might be slight, so that she would recover anyway, or so severe that another form of communication might be the only solution. Without a thorough investigation and the support of relevant professionals such a plan is doomed to failure.

In order to be sure that the client has the necessary skills to succeed in reaching desirable goals it is vital that some form of investigation as outlined in this chapter is undertaken, together with the gathering of all relevant information regarding that particular individual.

It is important at this point to stress the desirability of parallel planning and intervention. In the past it has been the practice amongst the differing professions to provide assessments and interventions on an exclusive basis without passing on information to others. Each separate discipline guarded its own system and resources, and regarded other approaches as alternatives. If the person is not to be swamped and further confused by an assortment of individual instructions and possibly conflicting ideas, a team approach and parallel assistance with appropriate assessments and interventions running side by side should be the aim. Rehabilitation will be made easier if resources and information are pooled. As appropriate, medical and drug regimes should run alongside physiotherapy, psychological, occupational and social support. Speech therapy as required, and the help of relatives and friends, should be included in this team approach. The degree of useful intervention can be monitored. In this way a relevant rehabilitation programme can be employed to cover the major needs and to allow all concerned to remain in touch with overall progress (Verwoerdt, 1981; Wattis and Church, 1986).

REFERENCES

Albert, M.S. (1981) Geriatric neuropsychology. *Journal of Consulting and Clinical Psychology, 49*(6), 835–50

Birren, J.E. and Schaie, K.W. (1985) *Handbook of the psychology of ageing.* Van Nostrand Reinhold, New York

Blackburn, I.M. and Tyrer, G.M.B. (1985) The value of Luria's Investigation for the assessment of cognitive dysfunction in Alzheimer-type dementia. *British Journal of Clinical Psychology, 24,* 171–9

Brotchie, J., Brennan, J. and Wyke, M. (1985) Temporal orientation in the pre-senium and old age. *British Journal of Psychiatry, 147,* 692–5

Christensen, A. (1975) *Luria's neuropsychological investigation.* Munksgaard, Denmark

Goodglass, H. and Kaplan, E. (1972) *The assessment of aphasia and related disorders.* Lea & Febiger, Philadelphia

Holden, U.P. (1984) The case against standard test batteries. *Clinical Gerontologist, 3*(2), 48–52

Holden, U.P. and Woods, R.T. (1988) *Reality orientation: psychological approaches to the 'confused' elderly.* Churchill Livingstone, Edinburgh

Nelson, H.E. (1982) *The National Adult Reading Test.* NFER–Nelson, Windsor

Pattie, A. and Gilleard, C.J. (1979) *Manual of the Clifton Assessment*

Procedure for the Elderly (CAPE). Hodder & Stoughton Education, Sevenoaks

Satz, P. and Fletcher, J.M. (1981) Emergent trends in neuropsychology: an overview. *Journal of Consulting and Clinical Psychology, 49*(6), 851–65

Schaie, K.W. and Strother, C.R. (1968) A cross-sequential study of age changes in cognitive behaviour. *Psychological Bulletin, 70*, 671–80

Schaie, K.W. and Labouvie-Vief, G. (1974) Generational versus ontogenetic components of change in adult cognitive behaviour: a 14-year cross-sequential study. *Developmental Psychology, 10*, 305–20

Spiers, P.A. (1981) Have they come to praise Luria or bury him? The Luria–Nebraska Battery controversy. *Journal of Consulting and Clinical Psychology, 49*(3), 331–41

Verwoerdt, A. (1981) Psychotherapy for the elderly. In T. Arie (ed.) *Health care of the elderly.* Croom Helm, London/John Hopkins University Press, Baltimore, pp. 118–39

Wattis, J. and Church, M. (1986) *Practical psychiatry of old age.* Croom Helm, London/New York University Press

Williams, M. (1973) Geriatric patients. In P. Mittler (ed.), *The psychological assessment of mental and physical handicaps.* Tavistock Publications, London, Chapter 11

Wilson, B.A. and Moffat, N. (eds) (1984) *Clinical management of memory problems.* Croom Helm, London/Aspen Publishers, Rockville, Maryland

Woods, R.T. (1982) The psychology of ageing: assessment of defects and their management. In R. Levy and F. Post (eds), *The psychiatry of late life.* Blackwell Scientific Publications, Oxford, pp. 68–113

Woods, R.T. and Britton, P.G. (1985) *Clinical psychology with the elderly.* Croom Helm, London/Aspen Publishers, Rockville, Maryland

3

Mythology and Dementia

Una Holden

Over the centuries mankind's creative imagination has produced a wealth of strange tales and commonly held beliefs. The need to use imagination in this way has many reasons behind it. These include both honest and dishonest attempts to weave interesting stories, an embroidery to the deeds of heroes, efforts to make the unacceptable more tolerable, a justification of fear reactions or a means to convince others of the validity of a particular theory. The commonest reason appears to be an attempt to explain that which seems to be inexplicable. Man has always sought an answer from his limited experience, knowledge or consideration for all that he perceives by whatever means and sense this perception reaches him. Unwillingness to admit to ignorance, or laziness in seeking further information, leads him to trust his own inadequate resources. Quite frequently his finite abilities have proved insufficient to arrive at the truth, but sometimes his plausibility has succeeded in influencing others and so a widespread belief in a completely errone- ous story or concept has grown. What is remarkable about these myths is that they can be replicated in totally different cultures and travel an extraordinary distance.

In many countries, legends of a similar nature will be repeated. Heroes, with different names, battle with two-headed, three-eyed monsters, dragons or beguiling sirens. Family feuds lead to tragedy when young people from either side fall in love; land arguments are settled by declaring; 'The first hand to touch the soil will be that of the owner for evermore'. Innumerable hands from countries all around the world have been severed to found a dynasty, and so it goes on.

It was not just ancient man who created beliefs or stories

51

which were widely accepted. There is a society in present-day Britain which is attempting to trace the origins of the modern urban myth. Who has not heard of the friend of a friend who gave a lift to some woman with a case and who vanished after a mile, or of the dog, black of course, who walks regularly along a lonely beach and also vanishes, or even of that famous piece of Take-Away chicken that had an extremely long tail?

Medical myths

The history of medicine is studded with prime examples of unfounded 'truths' and practices. Many of these have become so embedded in the mind of the public that they are hard to eradicate. Unfortunately they are also accepted by far too many professional people as well! There are many examples, but the use of the expression 'Oh, she's just an hysterical woman' will serve as well as any.

The Greeks were responsible for this one. *Hystera* means womb. The old physicians believed that when a woman became emotionally distraught it was due to a 'wandering womb'. The treatment for this wandering was to use a form of smoke-bomb to persuade it to return to its proper place. Other gadgetry was devised later, horrendous to behold and doubtless even more so in its application, which was intended to frighten the womb back into place! This unspeakable treatment was used on unmentionable parts until comparatively recently. The chauvinistic Freud did nothing to discourage the belief, and added further fuel to the idea that only women became hysterical. As modern psychology has, at last, clearly identified that male 'hysteria' is as common as female 'vapours' the problem of the wandering womb takes on interesting dimensions!

Complicating the clarification of what is and what is not true is the fact that some old wives' tales are being found, by modern research, to have an element of truth in them. It would seem that fish *is* good for the brain, boiled onion water *is* good for colds, and for heart care the onion is valuable. Garlic was used to ward off witches, Henry VIII planted garlic to protect his roses from disease. Garlic has been found to guard against disease, even with roses, so it has proved good for the health if not for the breath. One day someone will find out why sleeping on a bed of horse dung was regarded as a cure for tuberculosis!

Definitions of dementia

Aretaeus, physician of Cappadocia AD 150, is reputed to have been the first person to use the word 'dementia' in relation to the thought disturbance of the old. '*De*' means damaged, '*mentia*' refers to thought. It would seem possible to apply such a term to a number of people who are far from old! After years of literature in which this word was variously defined there is now a reluctance to make any attempt to clarify the meaning. The subject is regarded as controversial and provocative, and has fallen into the category of 'subjects which cannot be discussed in polite society'. Books and articles are beginning to dodge the issue, become vague or mention only the observed reactions or lack of response associated with it. The 'dementia syndrome' has crept into recent literature without explanation. Older books and articles provide definitions which are so varied and diverse that no two can be found which can provide anything to suggest that the authors are referring to the same subject.

Some psychiatrists use a definition which roughly states that it is an irreversible, progressive and untreatable disorder associated with mental and social degeneration (Marsden, 1978; Gray and Isaacs, 1979).

Geriatricians talk about chronic or organic brain syndrome, a syndrome of global disturbance of higher mental functions in an alert patient. They also use the terms chronic or organic brain failure, persistent confusion, or senile dementia.

Neurologists regard it as a symptom or as a syndrome, characterised primarily by intellectual deterioration which might be due to a variety of underlying, or overlying, causes (Cummings and Benson, 1983).

The condition is seen as a particular pattern of behaviour. To the proverbial man in the street it could mean that someone was behaving in a 'mad' fashion — screaming, shouting and jumping about. To the professional it could mean that behaviour was odd and confused, that memory was poor, abilities were impaired and that daily living and cognitive skills were deteriorating.

To many people 'dementia' is a specific disease entity.

Global damage is yet another offering as a definition. This ignores the logical conclusion that global damage implies that the person is dying, dead or a zombie. Global impairment is a slight improvement, but strongly suggests that the investigations were limited and inadequate.

53

In view of this range of definition and assumption it is hardly surprising that the question 'what does it mean?' has been avoided, and any attempt to provide an answer regarded as a contentious subject. However, it is becoming imperative to face the problem and to find some more appropriate meaning for this nebulous concept for the sake of all those who are said to be 'suffering' from it. Most of this suffering appears more related to confusion over diagnoses than to the actual illness or disease concerned — whatever that might be.

Background and developments in knowledge

In order to examine the mythology surrounding dementia it is necessary to trace its history after circa AD 150 and to consider the research findings available at the present time.

Witchcraft has been associated with age for centuries. Even today children are taught to think of witches as old, haggard, misshapen women despite the evidence supplied by the media that modern witches and warlocks are of all ages and appearances. The poor old souls of yesterday who showed any signs of having a little chat to themselves, or of cooking up a few handy frogs or newts because they forgot to go to the butcher, got burned at the stake for chanting spells or mixing noxious brews!

Old folk of today who look a bit dishevelled and unkempt do not get burned as witches, but they are still liable to be 'put away' without proper investigation because the neighbours are convinced that they are 'crazed'.

The ancient expressions and expectations about age are still rampant. 'Old crone' and 'dirty old man' are referred to in conversation in company with many other expressions from the past. Society continues to build up prejudice and so influence expectations in the community which are accepted by the old as well as the young. 'What do you expect at your/my age?' covers everything from forgetting the reason for going upstairs, to having sex problems. In some communities sex after 50, or even 40, years of age is regarded as 'not nice'! This is probably the reason why older people or GPs will not attempt to solve such problems.

During the nineteenth and early twentieth centuries a large number of researchers, including Esquirol, Binswanger, Lhermitte and Charpentier, looked in detail at the question of the causes of dementia (Constantinidis, Richard and de Ajuria-guerra, 1978). The names from this period of study which remain commonly recognised today are those of Pick, Broca, Wernicke and Alzheimer. Abnormal cells in the brain were identified by many people, but it is Alzheimer's work between about 1907 and 1911 which is clearly associated with the finding of senile plaques, neurofibrillary tangles and granulovascular changes in the brains of younger people. This disease process was degenerative and referred to as pre-senile dementia or Alzheimer's disease until very recently. Several workers challenged the idea that there was something different about the dementia related to older and to younger patients, Constantinidis amongst them (1978). It would seem that the only difference is the second between the time a woman of 59 becomes 60 and that second of a man's life between the age of 64 and 65 years! However, because this difference is so well ingrained some professionals continue to insist on the difference and refer to Alzheimer's disease in the over-60s as SDAT — senile dementia Alzheimer's type. Yet another reinforcement of a myth!

Psychologists cannot claim to be free from the taint either. The early researchers on intelligence, in their eagerness to establish credibility, managed with their highly biased material to introduce an expression to the public which refuses to be extinguished — namely, the IQ. Not only is this relic in current use, but the impression that age equals desiccation has stuck. The early results from older testees were so poor that if placed on a graph to show how intelligence and age performed this older group were almost at the same level of ability as the unborn child — untestable! The testers, with great condescension, decided to add a few extra points 'for age correction'! As their efforts left a lot to be desired with regard to theory, construction and validity it is no mean satisfaction to the present generation of clinical psychologists working with the elderly to find that modern research is proving what has been appreciated in practice — normal ageing does not imply the dreadful loss first expected (Schaie and Buech, 1973; Schaie and Labouvie-Vief, 1974). In most cases verbal ability improves with age, as do many other vital facets of the intellect — providing there is no trauma. There are changes — many can be due to added caution, consideration of alternatives, or even an unwillingness to be put in an embarrassing position. The whole concept of test procedure is undergoing modification and rethinking. The irrelevant, demanding test batteries are being replaced by more relevant material (Holden, 1984). Diminishing intelligence is undergoing closer investigation, and the prognosis for the ageing brain is much more promising than has been believed in the past. This must be consoling for the elderly statesmen and women of the world, not to mention all the famous and not so famous old superpeople who are actively involved in art, drama, science, invention, authorship and everything else which enhances not only their own lives but those of everyone else as well.

As results from the National Census data are released from time to time certain figures are incorporated into medical and other reports (Royal College of Physicians Report, 1981). The information given most prominence is that which reinforces the idea that age is synonymous with dependency, 'dementia' destitution and disintegration. The nation's resources will be drained by these growing numbers! The more positive aspects of these in-depth investigations seem to be filed away and forgotten (Craig, 1983). The fact that the incidence or prevalence of 'dementia' is on the decline is conveniently ignored (Hagnell, Lanke, Rorsman and Ojesjo, 1981) or for some reason cannot be accepted. These figures are also kept quiet and given no publicity. Undoubtedly a similar pattern will be found in America, Europe and Australia.

Scientific research is as responsible for the proliferation of myths as anything else. Brain cells are widely believed to be lost from the age of 21 years at the rate of 100,000 a day (Brody, 1955). It is hard to clarify the full story behind this notion — as it is in the case of most myths. However, it would seem to have first surfaced in the middle of the nineteenth century and is in some way associated with a beekeeping, pseudo-neuropathologist called Hodge. This gentleman is said to have studied his 40 bees whilst also being in possession of a few unwanted human brains which he had in his laboratory. His logical approach was to deduce that the bees' cells were burnt out by overwork, so by comparison the burnout in the human brain would be of a much more prolonged but similar nature. Researchers have frequently stated their concern about employing rat and monkey brains as a basis for human brain theory, but to use bees!

Despite early disbelief in such a possibility, neurones have been counted for some years now (Ball, 1977). Apparently man is born with a redundancy of neurones — those which are not built into a system or given a specific function can die out. On the developmental level continued loss, or the degree of actual loss, remains contentious. Earlier investigators could find no natural, or only minimal, loss of neurones over the years (Konigsmarck and Murphy, 1970; Corseillis, 1979). Recent studies tend to confirm minimal loss in healthy brains. Since the 1970s the literature has been full of sparkling arguments and neuronal counts and recounts in many areas of the brain. After much excitement there now appears to be a lull, and a general agreement that if there is any neuronal loss in normal ageing it is a modest one, and that even neurotransmitters and neuropep-tides are little changed (Bondareff, 1983; Wilcock and Esiri, 1983; Rossor, Iverson, Reynolds, Mountjoy and Roth, 1984). Disease and trauma obviously provide a different story and cause losses (Bowen and Davison, 1980; Mann and Yates, 1983).

In view of the statement by Boulding (1981) pointing out that only 10 per cent of the brain is used anyway, loss does not seem to be that important. Boulding notes that there are 10 billion neurones capable of being on or off, or of taking on different functions. If this is true then it would add support to the claims of the therapists who are involved in retraining and, perhaps, reorganising brain functions. With that many neurones about and willing to work the potential for discovery on the part of researchers, and rediscovery on the part of the patient, would be considerable.

Other interesting developments in the argument about brain plasticity come from the work of Buell and Coleman (1981). They have demonstrated that regeneration of brain cells occurs in old as well as young brains. This was regarded as a myth! Equally interesting is that such growth does not occur in patients with Alzheimer's disease. There is a long way to go before all these new findings can be clarified and made use of clinically. There is obviously much more to uncover. The door has been opened and at long last questions are being asked and answers provided. The long-accepted theories and common-place statements are being examined. Do enlarged ventricles really imply degeneration (Hubbard and Anderson, 1981), is there real brain atrophy and is there any relevance in brain weight or size (Naguib and Levy, 1982)? It is, perhaps, more relevant and logical to consider the effects of health care, nutri-tion and the general standard of living on the young of today in comparison with the young of 50–60 years ago. As the youth of the 1980s are, on the whole, bigger than the people of the earlier part of the century it does seem reasonable to expect that there is a difference in brain weight and size too, and equally a variation from individual to individual.

DEMENTIA IN THE 1980s

With the advent of new information and technology the excuse that further investigations could prove dangerous for the patient is no longer tenable. Full investigations should include elimination of the following before drawing any conclusions about the presence of a dementia-related state: acute confusion, delirium and depression. Confusion can be the result of many influences other than organic damage to the brain. Psychiatric, medical and neurological disorders can cause acute confusion or delirium, but emotional stress, excesses of drugs or alcohol, toxic gases, even environmental changes can affect a person's state of mind (Holden, 1987). With an old person the disorientation and clouding of consciousness due to physical illness can be mistaken for a dementia unless proper investigations are carried out. Equally the effects of strange environments and the loss of familiar things in familiar surroundings can precipitate behavioural responses which are similar to those of a patient with a dementia. When appropriately treated physical illness can usually improve or be cured.

The commonest error in diagnosis is the omission of depression as a possible explanation for the problems. The apathy, poor response and often unkempt appearance of the patient can lead the inexperienced to the conclusion that a deterioration process is present. Delusions may be present and there can be disturbances in drive, appetite, sleep patterns and eating. Real symptoms can be exaggerated, and memory appears to be poor. When time is given to such clients, and they are encouraged to talk, it soon becomes obvious that they are capable of providing a much more coherent history than would be obtained from a person with a dementia. A good social history and consideration of the possible difficulties experienced at home will also throw light on the true situation.

The more careful screening for these alternatives has undoubtedly contributed to the fall in reported cases of dementia, and appears to be influencing improvements in the service to elderly people in general.

When asked what the commonest form of a dementia-related state might be, the majority of nursing or care staff could indicate that it would be of a vascular nature. The general population would be of the same opinion. They blissfully refer to 'hardening of the arteries' as though this explains everything. It is almost a matter of course to greet a stroke in the over-60s as a definite sign of dementia — recovery seems highly unlikely. Recovery *is* possible and global damage is not the invariable outcome unless, as stated earlier, the person dies. Cerebrovascular accidents account for only about 10 per cent of all cases where a dementia is involved (Blessed, Tomlinson and Roth, 1968). Such states are now known as multi-infarct dementias (MID) and are the result of a step-wise process (Hachinski, Illiff, Zihka, Du Boulay, McAllister, Marshall, Russell and Symon, 1975; Harrison, Thomas, Du Boulay and Marshall, 1979; Brust, 1983). A small stroke occurs, followed by a period of stabilisation or recovery, which may last a considerable length of time; another stroke occurs which may have similar or totally different neurological or neuropsychological consequences. The sequence can be repeated again and again until the damage is severe enough to require permanent care, though often the damage is not as severe or as widespread as suspected.

Obviously there are a number of different cerebrovascular accidents depending on the site of the stroke, and it is vital to recognise these differences in order to provide appropriate treatment (Strub and Black, 1981; Cummings and Benson, 1983). However, the issue here is to stress that a single stroke does not necessarily cause a dementia. Even a series of strokes may not result in global impairment, as many functions may be spared. What is important is the need to identify retained function because it is with spared, or only slightly impaired, function that rehabilitation and retraining can start.

The rag-bag diagnosis 'senile dementia' is no longer acceptable. The use of this term implies an ignorance about procedure, proper methods, new findings and the relevant diagnoses and treatments (Mayeux and Rosen, 1983).

Furthermore, several of the so-called irreversible states are proving to be treatable, or controllable (Cummings, 1983). Hydrocephalus can, under certain conditions and with the help of neurosurgery, be brought under control and the person returned to work or normal living (Benson, 1974; Schurr, 1983). The profound effects of alcohol which have sent many a patient to a long-term institution can also be reversed (Carlen, 1978; Lishman, Ron and Acker, 1980). New findings, the isolation of syndromes, better understanding of the neurotransmitters are appearing each week in the scientific literature (Simms, Bowen, Smith, Flack, Davison, Snowden and Neary, 1980; Rossor *et al.*, 1984; Bowen and Davison, 1983; Morar, Whitburn, Blair, Leeming and Wilcock, 1983). It is becoming increasingly difficult to keep pace with them, but attempts must be made to do so or the elderly will not benefit and attitudes will remain static.

Expectations are frequently the reason for the continued use of the dementia label. Observers can fear the presence of deterioration by misinterpreting the effects anxiety can have on behaviour. Methods which convince both patient and relative that the forgotten message or the burnt dinner is due to memory lapse, rather than progressive disorder, can lift a depression and improve a memory remarkably quickly.

Other states of a serious nature may, or may not, at this time respond to treatment or be reversible. Tumours can be removed, there is some control for Parkinson's disease — but Pick's disease and others such as transmissible viruses or spongiform encephalopathies (Gibbs and Gadjusek, 1978; Corseillis, 1979; Taub, 1983) are still serious problems. These are just some of the many 'illnesses' which are clustered together under the title of dementia.

The subcortical dementias (see Chapter 4) — or states as they should be called, are rarely noted. The persons perceived as totally forgetful and totally incapable of performing tasks are often merely suffering from an apparent deterioration. They have no real aphasia, apraxia, agnosia or true memory or ability loss (Albert, Feldman and Willis, 1974). The patient forgets to remember, is slowed down — the activating system is deactivated — and is suffering from anxiety. The stress of being dismissed as useless by those around leads to an unwillingness to try. Mutism is also possible, although real ability is preserved (Albert *et al.*, 1974; Benson, 1983). Encouragement and consideration are vital in the early stages so that the person can be given an opportunity to learn how to fight the problems.

Alzheimer's disease

Alzheimer's disease is the major cause of intellectual deterioration. It is not vascular in origin, though there is no reason why MID and Alzheimer's disease cannot occur together. Most of the investigations of dementia are centred on this condition and are throwing light on all aspects of brain function and impairment (Mayeux and Rosen, 1983; Cummings and Benson, 1983; Wilcock, 1984). Wurtman (1985) states that the essential point on which scientists are focusing is the need to identify the cause and to pose hypotheses which can be tested out. He identifies six conceptual models, though there are others (Wilcock, 1984) on which work has been completed or which is under way. Wurtman's concepts for further investigation are:

1. A familial cause due to an aberrant gene or genes which have yet to be identified. Seventeen per cent of the relatives of Alzheimer patients have themselves developed the disease by the age of 80 years. Familial Alzheimer's disease (FAD) has been studied by Breitner and Folstein (1984), who provide a useful questionnaire. They suggest that FAD is closely linked with apraxia and language disorder.

2. The growth of abnormal protein structures as first isolated by Alzheimer — neurofibrillary tangles, amyloid surrounding and invading blood vessels, and amyloid plaques. Plaques alone cannot be associated with Alzheimer's disease, and occur in normal brains. It is the proliferation of these protein structures in specific areas, such as the hippocampus, which is associated with the disease.

3. Infectious agents — slow or transmissible viruses may not be viruses at all, but odd sorts of protein called prions. Recent work suggests genetic sources which may effect transmission (Baker, Ridley and Crow, 1985). Although there may be relevance to other states, transmission does not appear relevant to Alzheimer's disease.

4. Toxins — zinc or aluminium salts from water, tins, utensils or from dialysis programmes. This has been a popular hypothesis for some years, but until very recently there has been little evidence to show toxins influence the appearance of Alzheimer's disease. Recent findings are suggesting that there is a link.

5. Blood flow — Wurtman cites studies which show that

61

changes occur in youth in the methods whereby oxygen is released to the brain. The work suggests that in some people these changes do not occur, and as a result blood flow in later years is impaired with this group of people. The theory is vague and is not yet highlighted by any similar research.

6. Inadequate neurotransmitter systems — this is the most popular and researched concept. By the mid-1970s Alzheimer patients were being fed a diet of fish or a fishy-smelling concoction — the plant food of South American centigenarians — lecithin — in the hope that it would help the production of acetylcholine and related enzymes. The cholinergic system has relationships with memory and cognition and it seems certain, with Alzheimer's disease (Bowen, Smith, White and Davison, 1976; Simms *et al.*, 1980; Wilcock, 1984). Unfortunately, despite many attempts there has been little success in increasing the supply or improving memory. The work in this field remains active and exciting, and doubtless in time there will be a breakthrough. Different schools produce findings which either confirm or contradict previous work and so stimulate further enquiry. What seems certain is that Alzheimer's disease is *not* an acceleration of the ageing process, that normal brains are not losing any cells in great numbers or having problems in producing neurotransmitters. Deficits in the cholinergic–noradrenergic systems, and changes in other neurotransmitters or neuropeptides, are closely associated with Alzheimer's disease. Literally under the microscope are gamma-aminobutyric acid systems (GABA), serotonin, dopamine, the neuropeptides and even unknowns (Rossor *et al.*, 1984).

Furthering the argument about presenile dementia differing from dementia is an interesting finding showing differences between those developing Alzheimer's disease under and over *80* years of age. The over-80s have deficits isolated to the temporal and hippocampal areas with an insignificant loss of neurones. The under-80s appear to have a massive loss of neurones and neurotransmitters of a widespread nature (Bondareff, 1983; Wilcock and Esiri, 1983; Rossor *et al.*, 1984).

It would seem that the parts are being identified, but the whole is still being seen as through a glass darkly. Until Alzheimer's disease is fully understood it will be hard to find an immediate answer to each case — if this can ever be possible. Clarification is needed not only about causes but also about the diverse presentations clinically. At present memory loss, apraxias, aphasias, disorientations and even perceptual disorders are all lumped together in a manner which does not appear appropriate. In a recent review all the various attempts to delineate subtypes were gathered together (Jorm, 1985). Despite a careful analysis the article concluded that although Alzheimer's disease was accepted as variable in nature our present knowledge is insufficient to clarify subgroups, and longitudinal studies are required.

Several workers have identified clinical stages. It is generally accepted that there are three:

1. Slow insidious beginning. Usually memory losses and slight disorientation. Personality remains intact.
2. More memory loss. Disorientation for time, place and person. Silly errors in action or speech occur. Depression and anxiety may occur. Personality still intact.
3. Pronounced apraxias, disorientation and memory loss. Anomia common. Perseveration notable. Agnosia may be present. Acquired knowledge and personality impaired.

Obviously there is much variation, and differences depend on the area most affected. It does not follow that all functioning is impaired, or even involved. The *real person* is not submerged until late in the process. The situation should be thoroughly investigated and a surprising number of retained abilities will be found. It has been shown in study after study that even severely mentally disabled people can respond to stimulation; can relearn and regain more independence than was originally supposed (Holden and Woods, 1982/8; Woods and Britton, 1985).

Positive approaches

Efforts by health and social services staff to use positive approaches have resulted in a changed environment and atmosphere: one where things are happening and in which patients and residents are actively involved. The old custodial care system has no place in present society no matter how unconvinced are those who wish to continue along outdated paths. Wershow (1977) claimed that all the effort was only serving to help those working in a hopeless situation to feel that everything was not hopeless. He voiced the opinions of many, but events have proved all of them to be wrong. There *is* hope, and the answers are being supplied. While a multitude of questions await an answer there is already enough evidence to show the presence of change.

The active work of clinicians and therapists has led to the emergence of several approaches — reality orientation and its close relations reminiscence, milieu therapy, group living, and environmental modification (Holden and Woods 1982/8), not to mention cognitive therapy, family therapy and other psychotherapeutic programmes. All of these are making changes not only in the patients and residents but in the relatives and staff groups. The growth of relative support groups and volunteer organisations (Gilleard, 1984; Hanley and Hodge, 1984) — for example MIND, Age Concern, the Alzheimer's Society, Help the Aged, has had a role to play in making the public aware of the needs of old folk, and has influenced government policy and the support of the research work which is increasing the store of available knowledge.

Considerable gaps in knowledge among staff remain. The psychology of ageing is poorly appreciated generally. Countries all over the world are attempting to change this situation (Haugen, 1985; WHO, 1986) and attempts are being made to increase the number of trained clinical psychologists specialising in this field. But information and developments are taking a considerable amount of time to filter into practice. Too often explainable behaviour continues to be interpreted as a sign of 'dementia'. Hasty words, loose remarks and unqualified statements find their way into case notes. These give rise to false conclusions. Pejorative words include: aggressive, unmotivated, incontinent, confused or disorientated. The variety of meaning, interpretation and circumstance which prompt their use plays a major part in determining the implications. Unfortunately, notes rarely provide these clues. These biased terms can cause widespread and long-term effects which interfere with correct diagnoses, proper treatment and good relationships. Myths about an individual's behaviour are the common result.

In staff training one area in particular is poorly represented — neuropsychology. Behaviour of clients is often totally misunderstood by staff as well as by relatives and friends. It is important to consider brain function and the effects of specific forms of damage (Holden, 1987). Aphasia, apraxia and agnosia should be understood, and the possibility of explaining and managing behaviour in the light of this knowledge should be part of routine practice. If there is no understanding or awareness of the possible explanations it is hardly surprising that misunderstandings are rife and the belief in widespread 'dementia' reinforced (Albert, 1981; Holden, 1987). Retraining programmes cannot succeed if neuropsychological implications are overlooked.

Looking for logic

If all these facets of the situation are considered as an exercise in logic it becomes difficult to see dementia as a disease in its own right. How can a disease have so many variables? How can it be curable and irreversible at the same time? How can vascular disorders, brain cell losses or changes, and a host of unrelated problems such as tumours, viruses, alcohol effects, punch-drunkenness and so forth all fall under the same heading, or into the same category?

It is ridiculous even to attempt such an exercise, the premises are unconnected. If a person has a temperature the question — why? — is posed. Surely the same question is relevant when someone is showing signs of dementia? It is logical to ask — What is causing this dementia? To omit to provide a proper investigation of *all* the various possibilities and to quickly conclude 'Oh, it's dementia' is merely a sign of inadequacy on the part of the examiner. To regard dementia as anything other than a symptom is as puerile as elevating a temperature to the level of a disease. It has been referred to as a syndrome but, once again, the variability of the states, other symptoms and potential outcomes make the use of this term questionable too. One reason for the continued vagueness surrounding the words dementia and confusion is due to teaching staff lacking the relevant knowledge (Holden, 1987).

Like other symptoms or signs dementia can be present in several forms. In essence it shows disturbances in cognitive functions, in daily living and social behaviours. According to the true cause, the source of the problem and the area affected, differences in presentation will be seen. One person may have anomia, another spatial disorientation. It must be remembered that the brain is a complicated piece of machinery and damage or dementia, concerned with one part or function of it, does not imply that damage to any other part is certain to occur.

The findings from Sweden (Hagnell *et al.*, 1981) showing a drop in the prevalence of dementia are almost certainly reflecting the present enlightened climate. Improved diagnosis means that delirium and physical illness are noted, and that correct treatment is being instigated more frequently. In other words the *cause* of the so-called dementia is being treated where possible. Research has led to better identification of previously unknown or difficult-to-investigate syndromes, and so the diagnostic field of possibilities has grown. The availability of better training and transmission of knowledge has led to improved care and the use of positive approaches by all staff and clearer understanding by more relatives. When these innovations reach an even wider audience perhaps a 'diagnosis' of 'dementia' will vanish entirely and its prevalence as a symptom decrease even more.

Unfortunately, myths are hard to eradicate; at least one can always hope.

REFERENCES

Albert, M.L., Feldman, R.G. and Willis, A.L. (1974) The 'subcortical dementia' of progressive supranuclear palsy. *Journal of Neurology, Neurosurgery and Psychiatry, 37*, 121–30

Albert, M.S. (1981) Geriatric neuropsychology, *Journal of Consulting and Clinical Psychology, 49*(6), 835–50

Baker, H.F., Ridley, R.M. and Crow, T.J. (1985) Experimental transmission of an autosomal dominant spongiform encephalopathy: does the infectious agent originate in the human genome?, *British Medical Journal, 291*, 299–302

Ball, M. (1977) Neuronal loss, neurofibrillary tangles and granulovascular degeneration in the hippocampus with ageing and dementia. *Acta Neuropathologica, 37*, 111–18

Benson, D.F. (1974) Normal pressure hydrocephalus: a controversial entity. *Geriatrics*, June, pp. 125–32

Benson, D.F. (1983) Subcortical dementia. A clinical approach. In R. Mayeux and D.W. Rosen (eds), *The dementias*. Raven Press, New York, pp. 185–94

Blessed, G., Tomlinson, B.E. and Roth, M. (1968) The association between quantitative measures of dementia and senile change in the cerebral grey matter of elderly subjects. *British Journal of Psychiatry, 114,* 797–811

Bondareff, W. (1983) Age and Alzheimer disease. *Lancet,* June, p. 1447

Boulding, K. (1981) Human knowledge as a special system. *Behavioural Sciences, 26,* 93–105

Bowen, D.M. and Davison, A.N. (1980) Biochemical changes in the cholinergic system of the ageing brain and in senile dementia. *Psychological Medicine, 10,* 315–19

Bowen, D.M. and Davison, A.N. (1983) Biochemical assessment of serotoninergic and cholinergic dysfunction in cerebral atrophy in Alzheimer's disease. *Journal of Neurochemistry, 29,* 320–4

Bowen, D.M., Smith, C.B., White, P. and Davison, A.N. (1976) Neurotransmitter related enzymes and indices of hypoxia in senile dementia and other abiotrophies. *Brain, 99,* 459–96

Breitner, J.C.S. and Folstein, M.F. (1984) Familial Alzheimer dementia: a prevalent disorder with specific clinical features. *Psychological Medicine, 14,* 63–80

Brody, H. (1955) Organisation of the cerebral cortex. *Journal of Comparative Neurology, 102,* 511–56

Brust, J.C.M. (1983) Dementia and cerebrovascular disease. In R. Mayeux and W.D. Rosen (eds), *The dementias.* Raven Press, New York, pp. 131–47

Buell, S.J. and Coleman, P.D. (1981) Quantitative evidence for selective dendritic growth in normal human ageing but not in senile dementia. *Brain Research, 214,* 23–41

Carlen, P.L. (1978) Reversible cerebral atrophy in recently abstinent chronic alcoholics measured by computed tomography scans. *Science, 200,* 1076–8

Constantinidis, J. (1978) Is Alzheimer's disease a major form of senile dementia? Clinical, anatomical and genetic data. In R. Katzman, R.D. Terry, and K.L. Bick (eds), *Alzheimer's disease; senile dementia and related disorders.* Raven Press, New York, pp. 15–25

Constantinidis, J., Richard, J. and de Ajuriaguerra J. (1978) Dementias with seniles plaques and neurofibrillary changes. In A.D. Isaacs and F. Post (eds), *Studies in geriatric psychiatry.* Wiley, New York, pp. 121–54

Corseillis, J.A.N. (1979) On the transmission of dementia. *British Journal of Psychiatry, 134,* 553–9

Craig, J. (1983) Growth of the elderly population. *Population Trends,* Summer, pp. 28–33

Cummings, J.L. (1983) Treatable dementias. In R. Mayeux and W.D. Rosen (eds), *Advances in neuroloogy,* vol. 38: *The dementias.* Raven Press, New York, pp. 165–83

Cummings, J.L. and Benson, D.F. (1983) *Dementia: a clinical approach.* Butterworths, London

Gibbs, C.J. and Gadjusek, D.C. (1978) Subacute spongiform encephalitis: the transmissible viruses. In R. Katzman, R.D. Terry and K.L.

Bick (eds), *Alzheimer's disease: senile dementia and related disorders*. Raven Press, New York, pp. 559–76

Gilleard, C.J. (1984) *Living with dementia*. Croom Helm, London/The Charles Press, Philadelphia

Gray, B. and Isaacs, B. (1979) *Care of the elderly mentally infirm*. Tavistock, London

Hachinski, V.C., Illiff, L.D., Zihka E., Du Boulay, G.H., McAllister, V.L., Marshall, J., Russell, R.W.R. and Symon, I. (1975) Cerebral blood flow in dementia. *Archives of Neurology, 32*, 632–7

Hagnell, O., Lanke, J., Rorsman, B. and Ojesjo, L. (1981) Does the incidence of age psychosis decrease? *Neuropsychobiology, 7*, 201–11

Hanley, I.G. and Hodge, J. (eds) (1984) *Psychological approaches to the care of the elderly*. Croom Helm, London and New York

Haugen, P.K. (1985) *Dementia in old age — treatment approaches*. Norsk Gerontologist Institutt, Report 5

Harrison, M.J.G., Thomas, D.J., Du Boulay, G.H. and Marshall, J. (1979) Multi-infarct dementia. *Journal of the Neurological Sciences, 40*, 97–103

Holden, U.P. (1984) Assessment of dementia; the case against standard test batteries. *Clinical Gerontologist, 3*(2), 48–52

Holden, U.P. (1987) *Looking at confusion*. Winslow Press, Bicester, Oxon

Holden, U.P. and Woods, R.T. (1982/8) *Reality orientation: psychological approaches to the 'confused' elderly*. Churchill Livingstone, Edinburgh

Hubbard, B.M. and Anderson, J.M. (1981) A quantitative study of cerebral atrophy in old age and senile dementia. *Journal of the Neurological Sciences, 50*, 135–45

Jorm, A.F. (1985) Subtypes of Alzheimer's dementia: a conceptual analysis and critical review. *Psychological Medicine, 15*, 543–53

Konigsmarck, B.S.W. and Murphy, E.A. (1970) Neuronal populations in the human brain. *Nature, 228*, 1335–6

Lishman, W.A., Ron, M. and Acker, W. (1980) Computed tomography of the brain and psychometric assessment of alcoholic patients — a British study. In D. Richter (ed.) *Addiction and brain damage*. Croom Helm, London

Mann, D.M.A. and Yates, P.O. (1983) The ageing brain. *Geriatric Medicine*, April, pp. 275–81

Marsden, C.D. (1978) The diagnosis of dementia. In D. Isaacs and F. Post (eds), *Studies in geriatric psychiatry*. Wiley, New York, pp. 95–118

Mayeux, R. and Rosen, W.D. (1983) *The dementias*. Advances in Neurology, vol. 38. Raven Press, New York

Morar, C., Whitburn, S.B., Blair, J.A., Leeming, R.J. and Wilcock, G.K. (1983) Tetrahydrobiopterin in senile dementia of the Alzheimer type, *Journal of Neurology, Neurosurgery and Psychiatry, 46*, 582

Naguib, M. and Levy, R. (1982) Prediction of outcome in senile dementia — a computed tomography study. *British Journal of*

Psychiatry, 140, 263–7

Rossor, M.N., Iverson, L.L., Reynolds, G.P., Mountjoy, C.Q. and Roth, M. (1984) Neurochemical characteristics of early and late onset types of Alzheimer's disease. *British Medical Journal, 288,* 961–4

Royal College of Physicians (1981) Report on organic mental impairment in the elderly. *Journal of the Royal College of Physicians, 15,* 141–67

Schaie, K.W. and Buech, B.U. (1973) Generational and cohort specific differences in adult cognitive functioning: a fourteen year study of independent samples. *Developmental Psychology, 9,* 151–66

Schaie, K.W. and Labouvie- Vief, G. (1974) Generational versus ontogenetic components of change in adult cognitive behaviour: a fourteen year cross-sequential study. *Developmental Psychology, 10,* 305–20

Schurr, P. H. (1983) Hydrocephalus. *Medicine International: nervous system disorders.* Part 2(1), 31 July, pp. 1461–4

Strub, R.L. and Black, F.W. (1981) *Organic brain syndromes; an introduction to neurobehavioural disorders.* F.A. Davis, Philadelphia

Simms, W.R. Bowen, D.M., Smith, C.T., Flack, R.H.A., Davison, A.N., Snowden, J.S. and Neary, D. (1980) Glucose metabolism and acetylcholine synthesis in relation to neuronal activity in Alzheimer's disease. *Lancet, i,* 333–5

Taub, R.D. (1983) Transmissible viruses/spongiform encephalopathies. Recent data and hypothesis on Creutzfeld–Jacob disease. In R. Mayeux and W.D. Rosen (eds), *The dementias.* Advances in Neurology, vol. 38. Raven Press, New York, pp. 149–64

Wershow, H.J. (1977) Comment: reality orientation for gerontologists — some thoughts about senility. *Gerontologist, 17,* 297–302

World Health Organization (1986) *Dementia in later life; action and research.* WHO Technical Report Series

Wilcock, G.K. (1984) Dementia. In A.M. Dawson (ed.), *Recent Advances in medicine,* No. 19. Churchill Livingstone, Edinburgh and New York, pp. 57–76

Wilcock, G.K. and Esiri, M.M. (1983) Age and Alzheimer's disease. *Lancet, ii,* 346

Woods, R.T. and Britton, P.G. (1985) *Clinical psychology with the elderly.* Croom Helm, London/Aspen Publishers, Rockville, Maryland

Wurtman, R.J. (1985) Alzheimer's disease. *Scientific American,* January, pp. 48–56

4

Subcortical Dementia

Judith A. Peretz and Jeffrey L. Cummings

Dementia is a syndrome of acquired intellectual dysfunction involving several domains of mental abilities and resulting from brain dysfunction. Dementia is diagnosed when the persistent intellectual disturbance is acquired, not congenital in origin, and when at least three of the following mental functions are impaired: language, memory, visuospatial skills, emotion or personality, and cognition (abstraction, calculation, judgement, etc.) (Cummings and Benson, 1983). Once regarded as unitary disorders of brain failure, it is now recognised that dementias differ with regard to aetiology, pathophysiology, topography, neurochemical correlates, and clinical characteristics.

On the basis of clinical manifestations, two principal varieties of dementia can be identified: (1) cortical dementia characterised by loss of language abilities, memory and learning difficulties, and visuospatial impairment and presenting with aphasia, amnesia, agnosia and apraxia; and (2) subcortical dementia characterised by loss of functions such as attention, motivation, mood and arousal, and manifested clinically by slowing of information processing, lack of initiative, inertia, apathy, mood disturbances, forgetfulness and defective ability to manipulate acquired knowledge.

Traditionally, progressive dementia has been associated with neurological disorders involving primarily the cerebral cortex. Dementia of the Alzheimer type (DAT) and Pick's disease are the principal examples of processes whose most prominent pathological changes are in the cortex. In subcortical dementia the major pathophysiologic processes involve subcortical structures and mechanisms. Diseases producing subcortical dementia include: Parkinson's disease, Huntington's disease, Wilson's

Table 4.1: Classification of common causes of dementia

A. Dementia with predominantly cortical symptomatology
    Alzheimer's disease
    Pick's disease
    Multi-infarct dementia with cortical symptomatology
        Angular gyrus syndrome
        Multiple cortical infarctions

B. Dementia with cortical and subcortical symptomatology
    Jakob–Creutzfeldt disease
    Multi-infarct dementia with cortical and subcortical involvement
    CNS tumours
    Subdural haematomas
    Remote effect of neoplasm on the CNS
    Multiple sclerosis and other myelinoclastic disorders
    Post-traumatic encephalopathy
    Metabolic and systemic illnesses with CNS effects
    Toxic encephalopathies

C. Dementia with predominantly subcortical symptomatology
    Huntington's disease
    Parkinson's disease
    Progressive supranuclear palsy
    Wilson's disease
    Spinocerebellar degeneration
    Idiopathic basal ganglia calcifications
    Miscellaneous rare subcortical degenerative disorders
    Dementia syndrome of depression
    Hydrocephalus
    Multi-infarct dementia with predominantly subcortical infarctions

---

disease, progressive supranuclear palsy, and spinocerebellar degenerations. Other more rare extrapyramidal disorders also produce subcortical dementia, and the syndrome may also result from multiple subcortical infarctions as well as from infectious, traumatic and neoplastic processes involving subcortical structures. Table 4.1 presents a classification of the major dementia syndromes according to whether they have predominantly cortical or subcortical manifestations or have mixed cortical–subcortical features.

The distinction between cortical and subcortical dementia syndromes is not absolute from a clinical or anatomical point of view. In DAT, cortical cell loss coexists with subcortical lesions affecting the substantia innominata, locus coeruleus, and raphe nuclei. In Parkinson's disease the major pathological changes are in the substantia nigra, but the subcortical changes also involve the substantia innominata and there may be depletion of cortical neurotransmitters in some cases. Cortical and subcortical

71

dementia are best regarded as clinical concepts that correlate with the principal site of dysfunction in the central nervous system (CNS). It is the combination of the mental status features, temporal order of progression of intellectual deficits and motor system manifestations that help separate cortical from subcortical dementia (Caine, 1981).

In the initial portion of this review the characteristic features of subcortical dementia are compared to those of the cortical dementias, and the available information concerning the role of subcortical structures in human intelligence and emotional life are discussed. In the second part of the chapter the major disease entities that are associated with subcortical dementia are described. The conceptual and management benefits deriving from the cortical–subcortical distinction are emphasized.

HISTORY OF THE CONCEPT OF SUBCORTICAL DEMENTIA

In 1912, in discussing the disease that came to bear his name, S.A.K. Wilson noted that patients with subcortical disorders manifest behavioural alterations including cognitive impairment. While not explicitly formulating a relationship between dementia and basal ganglia dysfunction, the implications of his observations were obvious.

In 1974 Albert, Feldman and Willis proposed the concept of subcortical dementia. Their initial formulation was based upon the analysis of the behavioural abnormalities seen in progressive supranuclear palsy (PSP) — a disease usually associated exclusively with subcortical pathology. One year later, McHugh and Folstein (1975) described a similar syndrome in patients with Huntington's disease. The subcortical dementia syndrome as proposed by these authors consisted of: (1) a decline of cognitive functions and memory abilities; (2) an absence of features classically attributed to cortical damage such as aphasia, amnesia, agnosia and apraxia; and (3) personality changes characterised by apathy and inertia.

In 1981 Caine suggested that the dementia syndrome associated with depression had all the features of subcortical dementia, and Cummings and Benson (1983) noted the similarity between the dementia of extrapyramidal syndromes and the dementias occurring with multiple subcortical infarctions in the lacunar type multi-infarct dementia and with hydrocephalic dementia.

CHARACTERISTICS OF SUBCORTICAL DEMENTIA

Neuropsychological investigations have refined understanding of the features of subcortical dementia. The syndrome is now recognised to be characterised by: (1) disturbed attention and concentration: (2) slowness of mental processing; (3) forgetfulness; (4) cognitive impairment; (5) neuropsychiatric changes including personality alterations, mood disturbances and motivational impairment; (6) visuospatial disturbances; (7) absence of symptoms of cortical dysfunction such as aphasia, agnosia and apraxia; and (8) an associated motor disorder.

Attention and concentration

Alertness, vigilance and the ability to sustain attention are frequently disturbed in patients with subcortical dementia. Patients may perform inferiorly on tests of concentration such as digit span, digit symbol substitution, trail-making tests and serial cancellation tests (Pirozzolo, Hansch, Mortimer, Webster and Kuskowski, 1982; Bowen, Kamienny, Burns and Yahr, 1975; Pillon, Dubois, Lermitte and Agid, 1986; Reitan and Boll, 1971).

The ability to maintain or to appropriately shift sets is also impaired. Patients with Parkinson's disease and PSP perform inferiorly on tests of set shifting and maintenance such as the Wisconsin Card Sorting Test (WCST). To successfully complete this test the patients are required to shift sets and to attend to the completion of a task, a demand these patients often fail to meet (Bowen *et al.*, 1975; Pillon *et al.*, 1986). Bowen *et al.* (1975) found that levodopa therapy 'awakened' the patients and produced moderate improvement in their performance on the WCST.

Patients with bilateral or left-sided Parkinson's disease may exhibit disturbances in visual attention and cancellation (Villardita, Smirni and Zappala, 1983). Similar disturbances of visual attention have also been described in patients with subcortical haemorrhages involving the right putamen and/or thalamus (Mesulam, 1985).

Mental speed

Slowness of thought out of proportion to the severity of intellectual impairment is characteristic of subcortical dementia. Girrotti, Carella, Grassi, Soliveri, Marano and Caraceni (1986) found that patients with Parkinson's disease had increased reaction time to predictable and unpredictable stimuli during the 'off' phase of the disease and improvement occurred during the 'on' phase. Evarts, Teravainen and Calne (1981) compared parkinsonian patients with aged controls matched for severity of motoric slowing, and found that patients with Parkinson's disease had significantly slower reaction times indicative of slowed central operations; and Wilson, Kaszniak, Klawans and Garron (1980) found that parkinsonian patients are slowed when they scan short-term memory stores searching for recently introduced information. Once regarded as related to motor slowing (bradykinesia), cognitive slowing is now regarded as an independent manifestation of Parkinson's disease (bradyphrenia).

In PSP, Kimura, Barnett and Burkhart (1981) found that patients needed twice as much time to perform a task as normals; and Hart, Kwentus, Leshner and Frazier (1985) found similar results when testing patients with Friedreich's ataxia on a task assessing short-term memory. Slowed speed of information processing is one of the most pathognomonic features of subcortical dementia and may be related to altered central amine metabolism.

Memory

Patients with subcortical dementia are impaired on tasks designed to test recent and remote memory. However, if given an increased amount of time to respond, and if encouraged with the appropriate clues, the subject eventually produces the correct answer (Albert *et al.*, 1974). Thus, the memory impairment seen in subcortical dementia is best defined as exaggerated forgetfulness, unlike the amnesia found in cortical types of dementia and in Korsakoff's syndrome where learning does not occur and recall cannot be facilitated. Patients with Parkinson's disease usually remain oriented and perform well on simple memory tests. However, more detailed memory testing demonstrates deficiencies in the ability to learn and remember, and parkinsonian patients score inferiorly in comparison to normals on tests of visual memory, learning of superspan word lists, paired associate learning, tactile memory and recall of remote personal and sociopolitical information (Reitan and Boll, 1971; Pirozzolo *et al.*, 1982; Freedman, Rivoria, Butters, Sax and Feldman, 1984). Patients with Parkinson's disease and Huntington's disease are more impaired on recall tests and perform better on recognition tests (Martone, Butters, Payne, Becker and Sax, 1984; Butters, Sax, Montgomery and Tarlow, 1978). Impaired recall of remote information is equally severe for all decades of the patient's life (Albert, Butters and Brandt, 1981). These patients do not manifest the temporal gradient characteristic of Korsakoff's syndrome (Freedman *et al.*, 1984). Recently, Direnfeld, Albert, Volicer, Langlais, Marquis and Kaplan (1984) found that parkinsonian patients with greater involvement of the right side of the brain were more impaired on memory tests than patients with predominantly left-sided involvement.

Memory impairment in Huntington's disease is similar to that of Parkinson's disease, but the patients are more severely affected. Abnormal performance on tests of recent memory is among the earliest intellectual impairments in Huntington's disease. Caine, Bamford, Schiffer, Shoulson and Levy (1986) found that patients suffered both a verbal retrieval failure and an impairment of verbal recognition, whereas Moss, Albert, Butters and Payne (1986) found that their patients performed nearly normally on verbal recognition tasks but had difficulty with recall. They concluded that the impairment on the recall task may reflect a disturbance in the access to, or retrieval of, information rather than in the consolidation or storage of verbal material.

In cortical dementias the memory loss represents a learning disturbance with impaired storage of new information. Moss *et al.* (1986) compared patterns of memory loss among patients with DAT, Huntington's disease and alcoholic Korsakoff's syndrome, and found that all groups of patients were significantly impaired relative to normal control subjects. However, Korsakoff's syndrome patients, Huntington's disease patients, and normal control subjects lost 10–15 per cent of verbal information after a 15-second to two-minute delay, whereas patients with DAT lost 73 per cent of the material. DAT patients also responded poorly to cues, and were not helped when the test

75

was converted from a recall to a recognition task (Cummings and Benson, 1986). Memory abnormalities have not been studied as extensively in other diseases associated with subcortical dementia, but preliminary investigations reveal that patients with Friedreich's ataxia have slowed memory scanning, and patients with PSP are forgetful (Albert *et al.*, 1974; Davis, Bergerow and McLachlan, 1985; Wilson *et al.*, 1980).

In summary, memory disturbance is a cardinal feature of subcortical dementia. The memory does not appear to be a true amnesia and the deficit is best described as 'forgetting to remember' (Hecaen and Albert, 1978).

Cognition

A variety of additional cognitive deficits are found in patients with subcortical dementia. Category naming (also known as verbal fluency and referring to the number of members of a designated category named in one minute) is usually impaired early in the course of Parkinson's disease and Huntington's disease (Caine *et al.*, 1986; Lees and Smith, 1983; Girrotti *et al.*, 1986). Patients with Huntington's disease are impaired on Full Scale Verbal and Performance IQs of the Weschler Adult Intelligence Scale (WAIS) and on the Weschler Memory Scale. The subtests of the WAIS dependent on abstraction and concept manipulation are most severely involved (Boll, Heaton and Reitan, 1974; Butters *et al.*, 1978). Impairments on tasks such as copying and mathematics are found early in the course of the disease and cannot be accounted for by the relatively minor motor disturbances that the patients exhibit at that time (Caine *et al.*, 1986).

Similarly, patients with PSP are impaired on the WAIS subtests involving digit span, digit symbol substitution, arithmetic, similarities and picture arrangement (Maher, Smith and Lees, 1985).

Goldstein, Ewart, Randall and Gross (1968) found that patients with Wilson's disease scored inferiorly on the WAIS before treatment, and their performance significantly improved after penicillamine therapy. Patients with Parkinson's disease are similarly impaired. They exhibit abnormalities on the similarities subtest of the WAIS and have difficulty shifting sets, abstracting, sequencing, and categorizing (Lees and Smith,

1983; Reitan and Boll, 1971).

The cognitive deficits of the spinocerebellar degenerations have not been well studied, but appear to resemble those of other subcortical dementias (Cummings and Benson, 1983). Likewise, the cognitive impairments in idiopathic basal ganglia calcification have been shown to resemble those of other subcortical dementias (Cummings, Gosenfeld, Houlihan and McCaffrey, 1983b).

In summary, cognitive impairment is a common manifestation of the diseases that manifest subcortical dementia. The patients are most impaired on tests requiring abstraction and manipulation of acquired knowledge.

Speech and language

Language functions are relatively spared in subcortical dementias. Mild naming difficulties may appear, and there is impairment of verbal fluency. Comprehension and repetition are not impaired until the late stages of the diseases and paraphasic errors are uncommon. Huntington's disease patients may have diminished use of grammatical forms, and Caine *et al.* (1986) found that patients tended to list objects or sparsely describe stimulus pictures. Obler, Cummings and Albert (1979) described a patient with PSP who manifested abnormalities in word selection and inflection of verbal output.

Mechanical aspects of speech are severely affected in the subcortical dementias. Dysarthria is one of the most characteristic abnormalities of the syndrome. In the early stages the verbal output may be decreased in volume (hypophonic) and poorly articulated. With progression the verbal output becomes severely hypophonic and dysarthric, and in the end stages the patient may become completely mute (Cummings, Benson, Houlihan and Gosenfeld, 1983a). Mutism is also frequently reported in subcortical strokes and in other bilateral disorders of the basal ganglia (Cummings and Benson 1983; Rekate, Grubb, Aram, Hahn and Ratcheson, 1985).

Thus, patients with subcortical dementia commonly manifest speech disturbances. Language is usually spared; and when language is involved the alterations are unlike those of the classic aphasic syndromes or the aphasic disorders found in cortical dementias.

Visuospatial skills

Visuospatial abilities depend upon intact spatial perception as well as preserved perceptual-motor functions. Subcortical dementias are frequently associated with motor symptoms, and the majority of the tests used for diagnosing visuospatial difficulties require complex motor responses; thus it has been difficult to determine whether the assessed impairments are due to deficits in spatial perception or difficulties in planning and executing the required movement. In spite of these methodological difficulties, the majority of patients with Parkinson's disease, Huntington's disease and PSP have been found to have visuoperceptual impairment unrelated to their motor symptoms. Patients with Parkinson's disease fail to choose lines at an angle similar to that of a model; and, when their head and body are tilted, larger errors are made by patients than by controls in choosing a vertical axis. Parkinsonian patients also have difficulty in touching parts of their body corresponding to a body diagram, on route-walking tests and on tasks that require mental rotations (Boller, Passafiume, Keefe, Rogers, Morrow and Kim, 1984; Danta and Hilton, 1975; Proctor, Riklan, Cooper and Teuber, 1964).

Caine *et al.* (1986) found that when copying a figure, patients with Huntington's disease tended to omit details and distort relationships between component figures. Brouwers, Cox, Martin, Chase and Fedio (1984), demonstrated that patients with Huntington's disease are impaired on tests requiring orientation to personal egocentric space. However, they performed better than DAT patients on visuospatial construction tests (like copying the Rey–Osterrieth complex figure) and on tests involving manipulations of extrapersonal space (e.g. judging the direction of one object in relation to another object — Brouwers *et al.*, 1984; Bulens, Meerwaldt, Van der Wildt and Keemink, 1986).

In summary, visuospatial impairment is a common feature of subcortical dementia. The visuospatial performance of patients with Parkinson's disease and Huntington's disease is more impaired when manipulation of personal space is required. Visuospatial function of patients with DAT, on the other hand, is more impaired on tasks involving extrapersonal perception and construction.

Neuropsychiatric abnormalities

Personality

Personality changes are common in subcortical dementia in addition to cognitive impairment, speech disturbances, visuo-spatial difficulties and memory deficits. When Wilson (1912) described patients with hepatolenticular degeneration, he noticed that they became 'childish', 'docile', 'excessively emotional', lacked insight to their deficits and had poor judgement. Albert *et al.* (1974), describing a much older group of patients with PSP, noted that they became apathetic with occasional outbursts of rage. Huntington's disease is perhaps the best-known example of a disease that causes changes in personality and psychiatric disturbances. The personality changes may precede the chorea and the intellectual deterioration. Anxiety, irritability, mania, depression, alcoholism, hostility, paranoid states, chronic dysthymia and lability of affect have all been described. In addition, patients with Huntington's disease often lack insight to their disease (Caine and Shoulson, 1983).

Similarly, most patients with Parkinson's disease experience some changes in mental and emotional functions during the course of their disease. James Parkinson (1817) noticed 'unhappiness' and 'melancholia'. Apathy, excessive dependency, fearfulness, chronic anxiety, emotional lability and depression are commonly described (Mayeux, 1984). The patients become less involved in family and social affairs, initiate fewer interpersonal interactions and are more content with inactivity. On the Minnesota Multiphasic Personality Inventory (MMPI), Parkinson's disease patients show depressive tendencies, hypochondriasis and schizophrenia-like thought (Beardsley and Puletti, 1971; Hoehn, Crowley and Rutledge, 1976).

Post-encephalitic parkinsonism, a permanent parkinsonian state that followed the 1919–26 epidemic of von Economo's encephalitis, was associated with a wide array of neurological and psychiatric manifestations including depression, acute episodes of anxiety, obsessions and compulsions, mania, schizophrenia-like psychosis, apathy, somnolence and rage outbursts. Pathological studies demonstrated destruction of neurones in the midbrain, subthalamus and hypothalamus, again emphasising the importance of these subcortical structures in behaviour (Bromberg, 1930; Fairweather, 1947).

In subcortical strokes (usually those involving the vertebro-

79

basilar system) personality changes are very similar to those noted in subcortical degenerative disorders: apathy, hypersomnolence, withdrawal, flattened affect and paranoid ideation are seen. The behavioural changes often have an acute onset (Caplan, 1980) but may remain permanently (Trimble and Cummings, 1981). Likewise, subcortical tumours involving the brainstem, thalamus and hypothalamus may produce behavioural changes before increased intracranial pressure develops. Apathy, irritability, rage and somnolence are most commonly described.

Thus, apathy and inertia, conduct disorder and personality changes are common features of subcortical dementia. The correlations between the intellectual impairment and the behavioural changes have yet to be explored.

Depression

In addition to changes in personality, patients with subcortical dementia may develop affective disorders and schizophrenia-like psychoses. Depression has received the most systematic study of all non-cognitive alterations in subcortical disorders. Depression is the most common mental change in Parkinson's disease and can be expected in 40 per cent of the patients (Brown and Wilson, 1972; Mayeux, 1984). This prevalence exceeds that found in other chronic neurological or medical disorders with similar disabilities. The depression does not correlate with the severity of the motor impairment, and may even antedate the motor symptoms (Celesia and Wannamaker, 1972).

Affective disorders also appear in 30–40 per cent of patients with Huntington's disease and may include depression or mania (Shoulson, 1984). Caine and Shoulson (1983) found that 11 out of 37 patients with Huntington's disease (37 per cent) met diagnostic criteria for either major depression or dysthymic disorder and, as in Parkinson's disease, the severity of depression did not relate to the severity of movement disorder or motor disability. Schoenfeld, Myers, Cupples, Berkman, Sax and Clark (1984) noted that the suicide rate is four times higher in patients with Huntington's disease than in the general population. Depression has also been observed among patients with PSP, subcortical infarctions, Wilson's disease and spinocerebellar degenerations. In contrast, severe depression is uncommon in cortical degenerative processes (Cummings and Benson, 1986).

Mania is rarely observed in Parkinson's disease, but occurs in Huntington's disease, Wilson's disease and post-encephalitic parkinsonism. Cummings and Mendez (1984) brought attention to the fact that a majority of focal lesions producing secondary mania are located subcortically in hypothalamic and perithalamic regions.

Psychosis

Psychosis is closely correlated with dysfunction of subcortical structures. A high incidence of psychosis has been described in Huntington's disease, post-encephalitic Parkinson's disease, Wilson's disease, basal ganglia calcification, subcortical strokes, trauma, tumours and spinocerebellar degenerations.

In Huntington's disease, schizophrenia-like symptoms may occur at any time during the course of the illness. Symptoms include bizarre somatic and persecutory delusions, and there is little correlation between the severity of psychosis and the motor manifestations. Dewhurst, Oliver and McKnight (1970) observed psychosis in 51 of 102 patients, and Caine and Shoulson (1983) reported psychosis in 6 of 30 Huntington's disease patients.

Psychosis is rare in idiopathic Parkinson's disease, and when it occurs it is usually associated with levodopa or anticholinergic treatment. Psychosis was frequently described in post-encephalitic Parkinson's disease.

Approximately 50 per cent of all reported patients with basal ganglia calcification have a schizophrenia-like psychosis (Cummings, Gosenfeld, Houlihan and McCaffrey, 1983b). Similarly, psychosis is reported in association with Wilson's disease, spinocerebellar degeneration and subcortical strokes and tumours (Goldstein et al., 1968; Trimble and Cummings, 1981). Recently, Cummings (1985) reported that patients with cortical dementia (DAT) had more severe dementia and manifested simple paranoid misbeliefs, whereas patients with subcortical dementia had less severe intellectual alterations and tended to have more complex and highly structured delusions.

In summary, affective disorders and schizophrenia-like symptoms are not infrequently associated with subcortical dementia. It seems likely that the same pathophysiological processes are involved in producing the intellectual deficits, the neuropsychiatric abnormalities and the motor disturbances of these basal ganglionic disorders.

Comment and contrast with cortical dementias

Behaviour depends on two aspects of neuropsychological organisation. The first includes rate of information processing, motivation, ability to manipulate knowledge, set maintenance and shifting, attention and mood. These are called the 'fundamental' aspects of behaviour. The other realm of neuropsychological function deals with the instruments for executing behaviour. Such 'instrumental' functions include communication, perception and praxis. Subcortical dementia produces impairments affecting primarily the fundamental domain: patients manifest psychomotor retardation, poor problem-solving, deterioration in abstracting and concept formation, dilapidation of cognitive functions, forgetfulness and motor disturbances. Instrumental functions, on the contrary, are preserved until relatively late in the course of the diseases. Patients with cortical dementia have their greatest impairments in the instrumental domain: language, praxis and memory are affected early. Patients produce a fluent, paraphasic, empty verbal output with impaired comprehension (aphasia). They have difficulties in learning new material and, when tested, cueing and recognition paradigms do not help (amnesia). Patients with cortical dementias have difficulties performing constructional tasks and are more impaired than subcortical dementia patients on abstraction and calculation tasks. Apraxia and agnosia may appear as the diseases progress. The most characteristic feature of subcortical dementia is psychomotor retardation, whereas the most characteristic clinical aspect of cortical dementia is aphasia.

Another dramatic difference between these two types of dementias lies in the almost total absence of basic neurological abnormalities in cortical dementias in contrast to the profound motor disturbances of the subcortical processes. With the exception of mental status examination, the neurological assessment is often normal until the advanced stages of cortical diseases. These patients stand erect, walk without hesitation, are agile and have no abnormalities of speech volume or articulation. Patients with subcortical dementia suffer from severe neurological abnormalities including changes in muscle tone (rigidity or hypotonia), involuntary movements and slowing of motor activities (bradykinesia), and dysarthria.

DISEASES MANIFESTING SUBCORTICAL DEMENTIA

Parkinson's disease

Idiopathic Parkinson's disease (PD) (also known as paralysis agitans) is a degenerative brain disorder usually becoming manifest between 50 and 65 years of age and affecting primarily the pigmented nuclei of the brainstem. PD has a prevalence of 90–180/100,000 population and an incidence of approximately 20/100,000 population per year (McDowell, Lee and Sweet, 1978). A predominance of men is evident among the victims of PD. With treatment, survival for 10–15 years after onset is common, and longevity may not be reduced.

Clinical features

The cardinal features of PD are tremor, rigidity, bradykinesia and loss of postural and righting reflexes. The classic tremor is a four to six cycle/second resting tremor that nearly always affects the hands and may involve the legs, head, and jaw. In some cases an eight to twelve cycle/second action tremor occurs in addition to, or instead of, the resting tremor. Approximately 20 per cent of cases manifest little or no tremor (McDowell *et al.*, 1978). The rigidity of PD may be of the 'plastic' type present continuously throughout an active or passive movement; or a 'cogwheel' or 'rachet' character may be imparted by superimposition of tremor mechanisms on the underlying rigidity (Lance, Schwab and Peterson, 1963). Bradykinesia is the most disabling clinical feature of PD. Manifestations of bradykinesia include loss of facial expression ('masked facies') with diminished expression, widened palpebral fissures and reduction of blinking; loss of gesture; micrographia; drooling; loss of associated movements (i.e. diminished arm swing while walking); and hypophonia of the voice. Postural and righting abnormalities include disequilibrium, difficulty recovering when jolted from their centre of gravity, forward bowing of neck and upper thoracic spine, flexion of legs and arms, and a festinating gait with small stride length.

Other clinical alterations that may occur in PD include loss of upgaze and convergence movements and autonomic dysfunction such as impotence, constipation and orthostatic hypotension.

83

Pathology

Histologically, the substantia nigra is the nuclear structure most involved in PD (Table 4.2). There is extensive cell loss, and Lewy bodies may be seen in the cytoplasm of remaining neurones. The principal projections from the substantia nigra are upward to the putamen and caudate, and in PD these basal ganglionic structures are deprived of the normal inhibitory input from the nigral neurones. Cell loss also occurs in the ventral tegmental area, a region immediately ventral to the substantia nigra. These neurones project to mesolimbic structures (amygdala, septal nuclei) and neocortical regions (cingulate gyrus, orbitofrontal cortex), and involvement of these neuronal projections may account for a portion of the behavioural symptomatology of PD (Javoy-Agid and Agid, 1980). Other pigmented brainstem nuclei including the locus coeruleus and dorsal vagal nucleus, are also involved in the degenerative process of PD (Greenfield and Bosanquet, 1953).

The most significant neurochemical alteration identified in PD is the profound depletion of dopamine and related enzymes from the substantia nigra, ventral tegmental area, caudate nucleus, and putamen (Table 4.3). Dopamine reductions of 90 per cent are noted in the substantia nigra at autopsy, and the

Table 4.2: Anatomical regions involved in disorders with subcortical dementia

Anatomical structure	HD	PD	PSP	WD	SCD	MID
Caudate	+	±	−	+	±	+
Putamen	+	±	±	+	±	±
Globus pallidus	+	±	+	+	±	±
Thalamus	+	−	±	±	−	±
Substantia nigra	−	+	+	−	±	±
Ventral tegmental area	−	+	+	±	−	±
Red nucleus	−	−	+	±	−	±
Locus coeruleus	−	+	±	−	−	−
Subthalamic nuclei	±	−	+	+	−	±
Substantia innominata	−	+	±	−	−	−
Cerebellar nuclei	−	−	+	+	+	±
Cerebral cortex	±	±	−	−	−	±
Subcortical white matter	−	−	±	±	−	+
Spinal cord	−	−	−	−	±	−

HD — Huntington's disease; PD — Parkinson's disease; PSP — progressive supranuclear palsy; WD — Wilson's disease; SCD — spinocerebellar degenerations; MID — multi-infarct dementia.

Routinely involved, +; inconsistent involvement, ±; usually uninvolved, −.

caudate and putamen have 30–40 per cent less dopamine content than normal. In addition to the dopaminergic system involvement, PD patients have less noradrenaline, serotonin, glutamic acid decarboxylase (a gamma-aminobutyric acid [GABA] related enzyme), and choline acetyltransferase (a cholinergic enzyme) indicating that non-dopaminergic neurotransmitters are also affected (Hornykiewicz, 1973; McDowell *et al.*, 1978).

Dementia

The dementia of PD is controversial in terms of its prevalence and nature. Parkinson (1817) contended that the intellect was unaffected, but Charcot and others soon recognised that dementia was a not uncommon complication of PD. Clinically overt dementia with disorientation, obvious memory loss, constructional impairment and deterioration in judgement, calculation and abstraction occurs in 30–40 per cent of PD patients (Brown and Marsden, 1984; Loranger, Goodell, McDowell, Lee and Sweet, 1972; Pollock and Hornabrook, 1966). More discriminating neuropsychological testing reveals, however, that compared to age-matched controls nearly all PD patients manifest some degree of intellectual impairment (Pirozzollo *et al.*, 1982). The characteristics of this ubiquitous dementia syndrome conform to the pattern of subcortical dementia: visuospatial skills, effortful memory, set maintenance and concept formation are impaired, whereas language, praxis and perception are spared (Albert, 1978; Cummings, 1986).

Table 4.3: Major neurotransmitters involved in disorders with subcortical dementia

Neurotransmitter	HD	PD	PSP	WD	SCD	MID
Dopamine	—	dec	inc	—	UN	±
Noradrenaline	—	dec	—	—	UN	±
Serotonin	—	dec or —	—	—	UN	±
GABA	dec	—	—	—	UN	UN
Acetylcholine	—	±	±	—	UN	UN
Glutamic acid	inc	—	inc	—	UN	UN
Somatostatin	inc	dec	—	—	UN	UN

dec = routinely decreased; — = uninvolved; inc = routinely increased; ± = inconstant involvement; UN = unknown.

HD = Huntington's disease; PD = Parkinson's disease; PSP = progressive supranuclear palsy; WD = Wilson's disease; SCD = spinocerebellar degeneration; MID = multi-infarct dementia.

DAT may account for a portion of the dementias associated with PD, particularly those with severe cognitive impairment. Boller, Mizutani, Roesmann and Gambetti (1980) and Hakim and Mathieson (1979) found an excessive number of plaques and tangles in the cortex of some PD patients at autopsy and hypothesised a link between the two disorders. In addition, Whitehouse, Hedreen, White and Price (1983) found that PD patients have atrophy of the nucleus basalis of Meynert, a subcortical nucleus supplying cholinergic innervation to the cerebral cortex and involved in DAT. Perry, Perry, Blessed and Tomlinson (1977) confirmed that some PD patients with dementia have a cholinergic deficit similar to that found in DAT. In an epidemiological study, however, Heston (1980) found no increased association between PD and DAT, and the proportion of PD dementias attributable to DAT remains uncertain.

Treatment

Pharmacotherapy has replaced surgical thalamotomy as the treatment of choice in PD. Anticholinergics remain useful in the treatment of resting tremor, whereas rigidity and bradykinesia respond best to treatment with dopaminergic agents such as amantadine hydrochloride, levodopa, bromocriptine and lisuride. The dementia symptoms may also partially improve following treatment with dopaminergic agonists (Halgin, Riklan and Misiak, 1977; Meier and Martin, 1970). Unfortunately, PD patients with overt dementia are most prone to the development of toxic side-effects such as acute confusional states, hallucinations and delusions (Lieberman, Dziatolowski, Kupersmith, Serby, Goodgold, Korein and Goldstein, 1979; Sacks, Kohl, Messeloff and Schwartz, 1972).

Huntington's disease

Huntington's disease (HD) is an idiopathic degenerative disorder of the nervous system that was first described by Huntington in 1872. It is characterised clinically by chorea and dementia. The gene for HD is inherited in an autosomal dominant pattern with full penetrance so that a child with one choreic parent has a 50 per cent chance of developing the disease. It is determined by genes located on chromosome 4. Males and females are similarly affected. Sporadic cases occur rarely.

The onset of HD is insidious. The age of onset ranges from 20 to 45 years with a peak around 35 years. In about 1 per cent of affected individuals the age of onset is below 10 years, and Stone and Folstein (1939) reported a series of cases with onset in all decades up to the ninth. The average course from onset to death is 14 years. The worldwide prevalence of HD is five to ten cases per 100,000 (Hayden, 1981).

Clinical manifestations

The chorea of HD begins with grimacing and choreic movements of the fingers and toes. There is opening and closing of the mouth, elevation of the eyebrows and faulty speech articulation. The hands are involved in flexion–supination and extension–pronation movements, and the fingers move constantly. Dystonia and rigidity emerge gradually and motoric disturbances spread to the trunk and neck. This leads to dysarthria, severe inco-ordination, irregular lurching and faltering movements of the trunk, and an ataxic gait with a peculiar dancing quality. In the final stages of the disease, most patients are rigid and dystonic with limited involuntary athetoid movements. Ocular control is impaired early in the course of the disease with gaze fixation abnormalities and slowing of saccadic velocity. Vergence abnormalities, loss of smooth pursuit movements and supranuclear gaze difficulties appear in the more advanced stages (Shoulson, 1984). Muscle stretch reflexes are increased in one-third of the patients. The muscle tone is decreased during most of the course of the disease and increases in the late stages of the illness.

Nearly 10 per cent of patients with HD have onset of the disease in childhood and adolescence. These patients typically have prominent rigidity and dystonic features, minimal chorea, marked disturbances of speech and ocular movement, a high incidence of seizures, cerebellar dysfunction and rapidly progressive dementia. Death usually results from aspiration pneumonia in the setting of progressive weight loss and inanition, or is a result of a successful suicide attempt.

Dementia and psychopathology

Nearly every patient with HD manifests personality changes. Half of the patients present with psychiatric symptoms prior to the onset of motor abnormalities, and about half develop psychosis after the neurological manifestations are established (Pincus and Tucker, 1985). Personality changes vary between individuals and include irritability, anxiety, depression and feelings of inadequacy, violence, paranoid states, apathy and lability of affect (Caine and Shoulson, 1983; Folstein, Franz, Jensen, Chase and Folstein, 1983; Dewhurst et al., 1970; Caine, Hunt, Weingartner and Elbert, 1978).

A high incidence of sexual aberrations is also reported. Pathological jealousy, indecent exposure, homosexual assault, voyeurism, sexual coercive disorders and promiscuity have been described (Dewhurst et al., 1970).

Affective disorders appear in 30–40 per cent of patients (Shoulson, 1984) and may be manifested as major depression, mania or alternating periods of mania and depression. The reported increased frequency of suicide among patients with HD correlates with the prevalence of depression and occurs early in the course of the illness in more than half of the cases (Rosenbaum, 1941; Schoenfeld et al., 1984).

Schizophrenia-like symptoms are not uncommon. The patient may manifest delusions of persecution or grandiosity. Hallucinations are also frequent and were noted by half of the patients described by Rosenbaum (1941).

Dementia with subcortical features is a constant finding in patients with HD. The cognitive impairment develops gradually with memory deficits and decreased verbal fluency appearing first. The memory abnormalities are more apparent when recall rather than recognition test paradigms are employed (Butters et al., 1978; Martone, et al., 1984). The impairment on recall tasks may reflect a disturbance in retrieval of information rather than consolidation of stimulus material (Moss et al., 1986). HD patients exhibit equal difficulties in retrieving information from the recent and remote past, and do not manifest the retrograde amnesia with temporal gradient typical of patients with Korsakoff's syndrome (Martone et al., 1984).

When testing for language abilities in HD patients one does not find paraphasic errors, but the patients show decreased verbal output and diminished use of grammatical forms. Mild low-frequency naming difficulties and impaired repetition may also occur (Caine et al., 1986). Whereas language is relatively spared, speech is markedly abnormal. Choreiform movements often involve the lips and tongue, disrupting pronunciation and articulation. Diaphragmatic movements disturb speech volume, rate, spacing and phrase length, and impart an explosive quality to speech output.

HD patients also evidence abnormalities of constructions and mathematics. Visuospatial performances are impaired on tests that require egocentric spatial ability and visual discrimination (Brouwers *et al.*, 1984). As the disease progresses, concentration and judgement become affected. Patients have difficulty with organisation, planning, and sequencing of information, with initiation of spontaneous activity, and with organisation of information.

On the WAIS, the major impairments are seen on arithmetic, digit span, digit symbol substitution, and picture arrangement subtests.

Laboratory evaluation

Routine serum, urine and cerebrospinal fluid (CSF) studies are usually normal in HD. Analysis of CSF transmitters and metabolites may reveal decreased levels of GABA and homovanillic acid. EEG is normal in asymptomatic patients and becomes abnormal with low voltage and poorly developed alpha rhythms in symptomatic patients (Kiloh, McComas and Osselton, 1972). Computerised tomography (CT) demonstrates atrophy of the caudate nuclei with loss of the convex bulge into the lateral aspect of the frontal horns of the lateral ventricles (Figure 4.1).

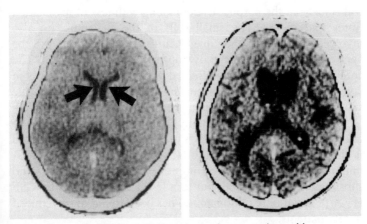

Figure 4.1: Normal CT scan (left) and scan from a patient with Huntington's disease (right) showing marked atrophy of caudate nucleus. Arrows (left) indicate location of normal caudate nucleus in lateral aspect of frontal horn of lateral ventricles.

Positron emission tomography (PET) reveals marked decrease in glucose metabolism in the caudate areas (Benson, Kuhl, Hawkins, Phelps, Cummings and Tsai, 1983; Kuhl, Phelps, Markham, Metter, Riege and Winter, 1982). Decreased glucose metabolism can be demonstrated before caudate atrophy is evident on the CT scan and prior to the appearance of chorea. Reduction in cerebral blood flow has also been found in fronto-temporal regions in patients with HD (Tanahashi, Meyer, Ishikawa, Kandula, Morte, Rogers, Gandhi and Walker, 1985).

Recent molecular genetic studies led to the discovery of a genetic marker (G8) localized on the short arm of chromosome 4. The G8 marker is linked closely to the HD gene and in 95 out of 100 cases it is co-inherited with it. Further investigations may provide a means of presymptomatic identification of the HD gene carrier, and may even provide a means of prenatal detection.

Neuropathology

Wasting of the head of the caudate nucleus and putamen bilaterally is characteristic of HD and is associated with moderate frontal and temporal cortical atrophy (Table 4.2). As a result of the caudate atrophy the lateral ventricles become enlarged and lack the characteristic lateral bulge created by the head of the caudate nucleus.

Microscopically there is disappearance of the small internuncial cells from the corpus striatum along with loss of myelinated fibres and gliosis. The small cells of the thalamus are also involved, reducing the microneuronal population of the ventrobasal thalamic nuclei by approximately 50 per cent. The cerebral cortex is variably affected with slight neuronal loss in layers 3, 5 and 6 and replacement gliosis. In some cases the subthalamic nuclei, substantia nigra and claustrum are involved.

The neurochemical defects in HD are only beginning to be understood (Table 4.3). GABA and acetylcholine are reduced in the striatum and pallidum of HD patients. Other neurotransmitters (angiotensin converting enzyme, somatostatin, and substance P) are reduced, but to a lesser extent. Recently CSF HVA (a metabolite of dopamine) has been found to be reduced in HD patients.

The basic pathophysiological defect in HD is the loss of small GABA-ergic neurones from the corpus striatum. These cells play an inhibitory role in motor mechanisms. GABA-ergic neurones are balanced with dopaminergic mechanisms originating from the substantia nigra as well as striatal cholinergic mechanisms. Loss of the GABA-mediated inhibition of dopaminergic cells results in motor disinhibition manifested clinically as chorea, athetosis and dystonia. Somatostatin increases striatal dopamine production (Uhl, Hackney, Torchia, Stranov, Tourtellotte, Whitehouse, Tran and Strittmatter, 1986), and increase of this substance leads to more abundant dopamine, and further contributes to the choreoathetotic symptoms characteristic of HD.

Treatment

There is no curative treatment for HD: it progresses in spite of effective symptomatic relief of the chorea (Shoulson, 1981). Major tranquilisers such as phenothiazines and butyrophenones, known to block dopaminergic receptors, best control the choreiform movements. The demonstration that GABA is decreased and somatostatin is increased in HD led to treatment trials with isoniazid, an agent that raises central GABA levels, and cysteamine, a drug that decreases somatostatin levels. Mild improvement of the involuntary movements was noticed with the former but not with cysteamine (Shults, Steardo, Barone, Mohr, Juncos, Serrati, Fedio, Tammingo and Chase, 1986). Levodopa and dopamine agonists such as transdihydrolisuride are useful in patients with parkinsonian features, but exacerbate the chorea (Bassi, Albizzati, Corsini, Frattola, Pioleti, Suchy and Trabucchi, 1986). The cognitive decline in Huntington's disease resists treatment. The psychotic and mood disturbances respond to treatment with antidepressants, lithium, neuroleptic agents or electroconvulsive therapy (Whittier, Haydn and Crawford, 1961).

Wilson's disease

Wilson's disease is an inherited autosomal recessive abnormality in the metabolism of copper that results in toxic accumulation of the metal in the liver, brain, eye and other organs. Deficiency in the plasma protein caeruloplasmin is a characteristic feature.

Hepatolenticular degeneration was described in 1912 by S.A.K. Wilson. He reported the clinical manifestations and pathological findings of a small group of patients who presented with rigidity, dystonia, contractures, tremor, dysarthria and emotional disturbances. The three autopsied cases showed extensive alterations in the lenticular nuclei of the brain and cirrhosis of the liver (Wilson, 1912). Wilson's report was of great theoretical interest because for the first time movement disorders and altered mental functions were linked to subcortical structures.

Clinical features

Two variants of the disease have been described: a juvenile type with onset in youth and relatively rapid evolution, and an adult type beginning between 20 and 25 years of age and following a more indolent course (Denny-Brown, 1964). Wilson's disease may present with neurological and psychiatric disturbances, hepatic dysfunction, haematological abnormalities or bone disease. Neurological abnormalities include rigidity, tremor, dystonia, inco-ordination, dysarthria, drooling, dysphagia and mask-like face. The central nervous system manifestations are almost always accompanied by the 'Kayser–Fleischer' rings. These are green, brown, or yellow deposits of copper in Descement's membrane of the cornea.

The juvenile type of the disease usually presents with mask-like face, dystonia, rapid finger tremor and choreoathetosis (Denny-Brown, 1964). The characteristic features of the adult variety are dysarthria, flapping tremor of the wrists, wing-beating tremor of the proximal arms and decreased blinking rate. Dystonic posturing is less prominent. Cerebellar symptoms are frequently present. Neurological disturbances are the first manifestations of the disease in approximately half the patients (Denny-Brown, 1964).

Wilson's disease presents with hepatic involvement less than half of the time. This may take the form of asymptomatic hepatosplenomegaly or acute hepatic cirrhosis. Thrombocytopenia, leukopenia and a Coombs-negative haemolytic anaemia may occasionally be present. Impaired renal function secondary to copper accumulation may cause various types of bone abnormalities. Renal tubular acidosis and Fanconi syndrome occur rarely.

Dementia

Altered mental functions were noted by Wilson (1912) as a manifestation of the disease. He described slowness, emotionalism, narrowing of the mental horizon, facility, docility and childishness. In addition, mental inactivity, impaired memory and poor concentration are prominent. Neuropsychological assessment demonstrates preserved language function and impaired abstraction and concept formation (Knehr and Bearn, 1956). The dementia may be partially reversible with treatment (Goldstein *et al.*, 1968).

Laboratory evaluation

The diagnosis is confirmed in suspected cases by the demonstration of either a serum concentration of caeruloplasmin less than 20 mg/dl and Kayser–Fleischer rings, or a serum caeruloplasmin less than 20 mg/dl and a concentration of copper in a liver biopsy sample greater than 250 mg per gram of dry weight. Most patients also excrete more than 100 mg of copper per day in urine, and exhibit characteristic histological abnormalities on liver biopsy. About 5 per cent of patients have a serum concentration of ceruloplasmin greater than 20 mg/dl. In these patients measurement of the ability to incorporate radioactive copper into caeruloplasmin is useful as a diagnostic test: patients with Wilson's disease incorporate little or no isotope into the protein.

Routine blood tests may reveal thrombocytopenia, leukopenia, haemolytic anaemia or hypophosphataemia. Urine tests reveal increased copper excretion and aminoaciduria, peptiduria, glycosuria, uricosuria and phosphaturia may occur. CSF studies are unremarkable, and EEGs may reveal slowing of the background frequency.

CT demonstrates areas of low density in the region of the lenticular nuclei in approximately 50 per cent of patients with extrapyramidal symptoms. The ventricles may be dilated. The brainstem may appear atrophic, and low-density areas in the regions of the dentate nuclei are seen occasionally. The areas of decreased density are not enhanced by infusion of contrast material (Nelson, Guzman, Grahovac and Howse, 1979). Patients without neurological symptoms may have normal CT scans. Presymptomatic homozygotes are identifiable by liver biopsy, and presymptomatic homozygotes and heterozygotes may have low levels of serum caeruloplasmin.

Pathology and pathogenesis

The lenticular nuclei of the brain are symmetrically atrophic and have a yellow or brown discoloration (Table 4.2). The putamen is more severely involved and in advanced cases may be cavitated. The white matter of the hemispheres, the dentate nucleus of the cerebellum, the globus pallidus, subthalamic nuclei and caudate nuclei may be involved.

The metabolic defect in Wilson's disease is an inability to maintain a proper balance of copper. Excess copper accumulates with pathological consequences for the liver, brain, eye and other organs. Death may occur from effects of copper toxicity in the central nervous system with little or no evidence of liver dysfunction, but in most subjects significant liver disease becomes apparent during the disease course. The liver has the characteristic findings of multilobular cirrhosis with necrosis, inflammation, fibrosis and bile duct proliferation.

Treatment

Therapy consists of removing the deposits of copper as rapidly as possible. The drug of choice is D-penicillamine, which forms a soluble complex with the tissue and serum copper and facilitates its renal excretion. Life-long therapy and a low-copper diet are required.

Continuous administration of D-penicillamine can reverse many of the symptoms of the disease and can prevent disease manifestations in asymptomatic patients.

Progressive supranuclear palsy (PSP)

PSP is a degenerative disease of the nervous system manifested by supranuclear ophthalmoplegia, pseudobulbar palsy, dystonic rigidity of the neck and trunk, and dementia. Attention was drawn to PSP as a clinicopathological entity in 1964 by Steele, Richardson and Olszewski.

Clinical features

Characteristically, the disease begins in the sixth decade (range 45–75 years) and progresses to death in 2–10 years. It is sporadic and occurs more commonly in males than in females (Steele, 1972). Diagnosis is based on a combination of supranuclear ophthalmoplegia, pseudobulbar palsy, axial rigidity, difficulty in balance, abrupt falls and change in personality. Initially, the neurological and neuro-ophthalmological abnormalities may be mild, taking a year or longer for the characteristic features to develop. Supranuclear ophthalmoplegia includes loss of volitional and pursuit eye movements despite relative preservation of reflex eye movements throughout most of the disease course. If the patient's head is moved in one direction the eyes will reflexively deviate in the opposite direction. Difficulty in voluntary downward gaze is a relatively early development, and when the patient attempts to look downward by leaning forward, his eyes deviate upward, further aggravating his downgaze deficit (Steele, 1972). This leads to difficulties in walking and frequent falls. Other neuro-ophthalmological abnormalities observed in PSP include microsquare wave jerks (small to-and-fro movements of the globes), saccadic pursuit movements, internuclear ophthalmoplegia, poor convergence, 'apraxia' of lid opening, and blepharospasm (Blumental and Miller, 1969; Ishino, Higashi, Kuroda, Yabuki, Hayahara and Otsuki, 1974; Mastaglia, Grainger, Kee, Sadk and Lefroy, 1973; Troost and Daroff, 1977).

Pseudobulbar palsy may also be prominent. The face becomes 'masked' and deeply lined, without expression; speech is slurred (dysarthria), the mouth hangs open and there is excessive drooling. The jaw jerk and the pharyngeal reflexes are exaggerated. Pseudobulbar affect with uncontrolled laughter and crying may occur but is infrequent (Behrman and Matthews, 1969). As the disease progresses the patients may become mute (Steele et al., 1964).

The extrapyramidal syndrome of progressive supranuclear palsy includes an upturned posture of the head, and marked rigidity of the axial musculature. Patients develop severe bradykinesia in the course of the disease, hence their superficial resemblance to parkinsonian patients. In contrast to the stooped posture observed in PD, however, the PSP patients are hypererect with neck extension. Tremor is unusual and, when present, it is usually an action tremor (Steele, 1972).

Dementia

Dementia has been regarded as an integral part of PSP since the first descriptions of the syndrome. Steele et al. (1964) noticed mild behavioural and personality changes in their patients; although only two of the nine patients originally described manifested severe dementia. The features of the dementia syndrome in PSP were later crystallised by Albert et al. (1974)

95

and became the pathognomonic characteristics of the subcortical dementia syndrome. The composite clinical profile of PSP dementia consists of: (1) forgetfulness; (2) slowness of thought processes; (3) alterations of personality with apathy or depression, irritability and euphoria, or brief outbursts of rage; and (4) impaired ability to manipulate acquired knowledge (e.g. poor calculating and abstracting ability). Language, a function highly dependent on cortical integrity, is usually unaffected. Apraxia and agnosia are also rare.

Neuropsychological testing of PSP patients reveals cognitive impairment with particular difficulties in carrying out tests believed to be sensitive to frontal lobe dysfunction (Maher *et al.*, 1985). Pillon *et al.* (1986) found that patients with PSP are more impaired than PD or DAT patients on tests assessing frontal lobe dysfunction. PSP patients also perform poorly on visual search and scanning tasks. This cannot be attributed to restricted range of vertical gaze of refixation deficiency and may be ascribed to central dysfunction (Fisk, Goodale, Burkhart and Barnett, 1982; Kimura *et al.*, 1981).

Laboratory investigations

Blood and serum studies yield normal findings, as do urine and CSF tests. EEG tracings are often abnormal but in a non-specific manner. Bitemporal theta activity and mild diffuse slowing are present early. With progression of the disease many patients develop bifrontal monorhythmic bursts of delta activity (Jankovic, 1984). Pneumoencephalography (now rarely used) reveals severe atrophy of the midbrain tegmentum and atrophy of the superior colliculi (Bentson and Keesey, 1974). CT scans reveal atrophy of midbrain, pons and cerebellum (Haldeman, Goldman, Hyde and Pribram, 1981). Regional cerebral metabolic rate for glucose, studied by PET, reveals a highly significant decrease of metabolism in the prefrontal cortex.

Neuropathology

Post-mortem examination discloses bilateral loss of neurones and gliosis in the periaqueductal grey matter, the superior colliculi, subthalamic nucleus, red nucleus, substantia nigra, dentate nuclei of the cerebellum and substantia innominata (Ishino *et al.*, 1974; Steele *et al.*, 1964) (Table 4.2). The nuclei of the oculomotor, trochlear and abducent nerves may also be affected (Blumental and Miller, 1969; Ishino *et al.*, 1974). The thalamus and hypothalamus are involved only minimally, and the cerebral cortex usually escapes the pathological process (Steele *et al.*, 1964). The histological changes consist of granulovacuolar degeneration and neurofibrillary tangles that have a specific structure unique to this disease (Powell, London and Lampert, 1974; Tellez-Nagel and Wisniewski, 1973; Roy, Datta, Hirano, Ghatak and Zimmerman, 1974; Tomonaga, 1977).

Neurochemical studies show reduced dopamine and homovanillic acid concentrations in the striatum, indicating that the nigrostriate dopaminergic system is involved. Choline acetyltransferase (CAT) may be moderately decreased, suggesting that cholinergic neurones may also be involved (Table 4.3).

Treatment

There is no cure for progressive supranuclear palsy, but antiparkinsonian medication may yield some therapeutic benefit. Levodopa is sometimes effective in controlling the bradykinesia and rigidity (Parkes, *et al.* 1971; Klawans and Ringel, 1971). Improvement has also been reported with amantadine hydrochloride, lisuride, pergolide and bromocriptine (Jackson, Jankovic and Ford, 1983; Neophytides, Liberman, Goldstein, Gopinathan, Leibowitz, Bock and Walker, 1982). Methysergide was reported to be particularly effective for patients with dysphagia (Rafal and Grimm, 1981). Benzotropine and tricyclic antidepressants may prove useful in selected cases (Haldeman *et al.*, 1981; Newman, 1985). With progression of the disease the response to treatment dissipates.

Spinocerebellar degenerations

Spinocerebellar degenerations (SCD) are a heterogeneous group of neurological disorders distinguished clinically by progressive unsteadiness in standing and walking, along with impaired co-ordination of limbs. They differ in the nature of the associated findings, which may include peripheral neuropathy, lower motor neurone weakness, posterior column sensory loss, extrapyramidal disturbances, difficulty in ocular motility and dementia. Differential diagnosis between the various forms of spinocerebellar degenerations is usually not possible during life (Greenfield, 1954). The spinocerebellar degenerations are commonly classified into syndromes that affect primarily the spinal cord, syndromes that affect predominantly the cerebellum, and syndromes that affect both the cerebellum and brainstem. Friedreich's syndrome is an example of the first group, cerebellar cortical degeneration of the second group, and olivopontocerebellar atrophy of the third. Friedreich's ataxia and olivopontocerebellar degeneration are the best-studied syndromes of the spinocerebellar degenerations, and will be used here to demonstrate the characteristics of this group of diseases.

Friedreich's ataxia

Friedreich's ataxia is a degenerative disease of the nervous system that has two potential inheritance patterns. The more common type is an autosomal recessive disorder with onset at approximately 11 years of age. The second type is an autosomal dominant pattern of inheritance with an age of onset of about 20 years.

Clinical features. In many instances the disease manifests itself for the first time during recovery from an acute febrile illness or physical or psychological trauma. The course is one of gradual progression towards helplessness within 10–20 years. Ataxia of gait is nearly always the initial symptom. The gait is wide-based and the legs lack co-ordination. The trunk and hands usually become involved months or years later. There is severe inco-ordination of the trunk and oscillation of the head, and the patients are unable to maintain a stable posture. The ataxia worsens when the patient closes his or her eyes, depriving the brain of visual sensory input. Dysarthria of speech is the result of the inco-ordination of laryngeal and pharyngeal musculature. Kyphoscoliosis and foot deformities are common; they may precede or follow the other neurological symptoms. Additional abnormalities reported in Friedreich's ataxia include nystagmus, blindness with optic atrophy, deafness and vestibular dysfunction. Muscle wasting (amyotrophy) is usually slight. Muscle stretch reflexes are nearly always abolished and vibratory and position sensitivity are lost. Touch and pain perception may become affected as the disease progresses. Many of the patients suffer from cardiovascular involvement: myocardial degeneration, ECG changes, paroxysmal tachycardia, or congestive heart failure are frequent causes of death. Periodic hyperthermia, acrocyanosis and disturbance of sweating have also been reported.

Neuropathology. The most prominent pathological change in Friedreich's ataxia is degeneration and secondary gliosis of the posterior roots and posterior columns of the spinal cord, Clarke's columns and the spinocerebellar tracts. Degeneration of the pyramidal tracts occurs later. The lumbar and sacral areas of the spinal cord are most severely affected, a fact reflected in the severity of the leg and gait ataxia. Peripheral nerves may be involved, but the anterior horns and anterior roots of the spinal cord are usually spared (Table 4.2).

Pure Friedreich's ataxia does not involve supraspinal structures, but atrophy of the inferior olives, and basal pontine and vestibular nuclei have been described in some cases. Severe loss of cortical Betz cells, optic atrophy and retinitis pigmentosa may also occur.

Kark and Rodriquez-Budelli (1979) reported reduced activity of lipoamine dehydrogenase in eleven patients with Friedreich's ataxia, and concluded that the enzyme defect may be related to a specific clinical subtype of the disorder.

Olivopontocerebellar atrophy

Olivopontocerebellar atrophy (OPCA) is a term given by Dejerine to a heterogeneous group of diseases with involvement of the cerebellum and the brainstem but with sparing of the spinal cord. Two clinical variants of OPCA are recognised: a familial form with autosomal dominant or autosomal recessive modes of transmission, and a sporadic form. In the familial form the average age of onset of 28 years (range 23 months to 53 years) and in the sporadic form it is usually around 50 years of age (Berciano, 1982). The disease first becomes manifest as a gait disturbance with unsteadiness of legs and trunk. Dysphagia, dysarthria and inco-ordination of the upper extremities occur later. Parkinsonian signs and symptoms, spasticity, intention tremor and sphincteric disturbances may be noted, reflecting more widespread involvement of the CNS. Occasionally the disease may be complicated by ocular abnormalities such as macular degeneration, slowly progressive optic atrophy and supranuclear ophthalmoplegia. Myoclonus, involuntary movement or cramps may also occur.

Pathology. The principal pathological changes in OPCA are severe involvement of the inferior olivary and pontine nuclei, shrunken inferior and middle cerebellar peduncles, atrophy of the cerebellar white matter with loss of Purkinje cells, and thinning of the granular and molecular layers of the cerebellum (Netsky, 1968; Oppenheimer, 1976). The posterior columns of the spinal cord, the substantia nigra and the putamen frequently show cell loss and gliosis.

Recently, a biochemical imbalance in asparate–taurine concentration in the cerebellum of patients with OPCA has been described (Perry, Perry, Blessed and Tomlinson, 1977).

Dementia

Dementia with subcortical-type characteristics is a frequent, if not uniform, finding in this group of diseases (Cummings and Benson, 1983). Kark and Rodriquez-Budelli (1979) reported abnormalities in mental status in eleven of twelve patients with Friedreich's ataxia. Sjogren (cited by Davies, 1949) found that 58 per cent of patients with Friedreich's syndrome exhibited progressive dementia.

The nature of the mental changes occurring in these disorders has received little systematic attention. Reported behavioural changes include slow cognition, impaired memory, emotional and personality changes, slowed information processing speed, impaired concentration, poor judgement, confusion and lability of affect (Akelaitis, 1937–8; Carter and Sukavajuna, 1956; Chandler and Bebin, 1956; Hamilton, Frick, Takahashi and Hopping, 1983; Hart *et al.*, 1985). Dementia appears to be more common in families that manifest several variants of spinocerebellar degeneration, suggesting more widespread involvement of the central nervous system (Cummings and Benson, 1983). Neuropsychiatric disturbances reported in OPCA include schizophrenia-like psychosis, bipolar affective disorders and conduct disorders (Akelaitis, 1937–8; Berciano, 1982; Hamilton *et al.*, 1983; Shepherd, 1955). These disturbances may appear in any phase of the disease but are more common in the middle and late periods (Berciano, 1982).

Vascular dementias

Multi-infarct dementia

Multi-infarct dementia (MID) is a progressive deterioration of intellectual functions caused by the occurrence of multiple (small or large) cerebral infarctions. MID will be discussed as an example of a dementing process characterised by cortical and subcortical pathology (depending upon the site of infarctions) and accordingly manifesting a mixed picture of cortical and subcortical dementia.

The prevalence of MID ranges from 8 to 30 per cent of the total spectrum of patients evaluated for dementia (Beck, Benson and Scheibel, 1982). Post-mortem studies have revealed that, among patients with progressive fatal dementias, 50 per cent have DAT, 20 per cent have vascular dementia and 20 per cent have a mixture of the two (Jellinger, 1976). Recognition of MID is important because of its association with treatable conditions such as hypertension or recurrent embolisation (from cardiac or major cerebral arteries). Early recognition and treatment may arrest deterioration and permit some degree of recovery.

Clinical features. The term 'multi-infarct dementia' was coined by Hachinski, Lassen and Marshall (1974) to emphasise the fact that vascular disease may be held responsible for production of dementia only through production of cerebral infarctions, not through low-flow mechanisms without completed stroke. The clinical picture of MID is determined by the cumulative effect of the cerebral insults. The patients suffer acute focal neurological deficits such as aphasia, amnesia, apraxia, visuomotor and visuospatial disorders, paresis, dysarthria, dysphagia or inco-ordination. After the acute event there is usually limited recovery, but the patient may be left with permanent neurological and intellectual deficits. The course is often characterised by an abrupt onset and step-wise accumulation of neurological and intellectual disturbances. The extent of the intellectual impairment is determined by the number of infarctions, their size and their locations.

Damage to specific areas of the brain produces regionally specific deficits. Thus, an infarct may be cortical and produce 'cortical signs' such as aphasia (left hemispheric infarct in right-handed people), visuospatial difficulties (parietal or frontal

101

infarctions), agnosia (occipital or occipitotemporal infarctions), memory deficits (temporal or limbic infarction), or an Alzheimer-like syndrome (left angular gyrus infarction). Infarctions may be subcortical and produce memory deficits (thalamic lesions), speech disturbances (basal ganglia, bilateral internal capsule lesions), or mood and personality changes (anterior or posterior circulation occlusions). Patients with bilateral lesions will usually exhibit lateralised neurological signs and pseudobulbar palsy.

Patients with MID frequently have evidence of systemic and cerebral arteriosclerosis and the majority suffer from hypertension and cardiac or renal disorders (Birkett and Raskin, 1982; Hachinski *et al.*, 1974).

Laboratory evaluation. Serum and blood studies should be performed in every patient with MID. Anaemia and polycythemia are both risk factors for MID. Blood smear studies can help identify haematological disorders, and an elevated sedimentation rate suggests temporal arteritis or other inflammatory disease. If systemic lupus erythematosus (SLE) is suspected, serum antinuclear antibodies and an LE cell preparation should be obtained. Chest X-ray may identify a carcinomatous process, and cardiac monitoring may help detect and evaluate cardiac disease or a cardiac source of emboli. CSF studies usually show a mildly elevated protein level (Wikkelso, Blomstrand and Nordoquist, 1981), and can provide valuable information regarding treatable conditions such as neurosyphilis or other inflammatory and neoplastic processes.

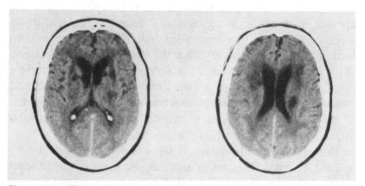

Figure 4.2: CT scan images of a patient with MID, shows multiple low-density areas corresponding to cerebral infarctions.

The CT in MID is characterised by enlarged ventricles and sulci, together with areas of hypodensity involving cortical and subcortical areas (Figure 4.2). Magnetic resonance imaging reveals multiple areas of altered signal reflecting infarcted regions of the brain (see Figure 4.3). Cerebral blood flow is reduced (Hachinski et al., 1975). On PET studies, MID patients have focal and asymmetric areas of reduced glucose metabolism. This is unlike the pattern seen in patients with DAT where hypometabolism is symmetric and spares the primary motor and sensory cortex (Benson et al., 1983).

Pathology. MID is a product of multiple cerebral infarctions involving the cerebral hemispheres. Several patterns of infarction have been identified, corresponding to the size and distribution of the intracranial vessels (Table 4.2). The most common pathological substrate of MID is lacunar state. Lacunes are infarctions 0.5–15 mm in diameter and located in the deep hemispheric structures, including the basal ganglia, internal capsule and thalamus. Involvement of the vessels penetrating from the cerebral cortical surface to the hemispheric white matter results in multiple white matter infarctions and ischaemia, a disorder known as Binswanger's disease (discussed below). Large vessel occlusion results in infarctions in the territories of the anterior, middle or posterior cerebral arteries or infarction of the border zones between these vessels when the carotid artery is the site of occlusion (Brown and Wilson, 1972; Fields, 1986; Hachinski, 1983; Hachinski et al., 1974). Brain infarctions are not additive, they multiply, so that further injury produces a cumulatively greater effect than the sum of individual infarctions (Fields, 1986).

Recurrent severe hypotension or repeated hypoglycaemic episodes cause damage similar to that of MID to cerebral structures (Plum and Posner, 1980).

The volume, as well as the location, of infarcted tissue contributes to the occurrence of MID. Tomlinson, Blessed and Roth (1970) found that mental deterioration was likely to be present if the volume of infarcted tissue exceeded 50 ml; and Kase (1986) argued that the critical amount of infarcted tissue was 150–200 ml. Below that volume the author found no clear evidence to implicate cerebral infarction as the cause of dementia.

Hypertensive fibrinoid necrosis of arterioles is the most common vascular pathology of MID. Atherosclerosis, infectious

Table 4.4: Classification of principal aetiologies of MID

Atherosclerosis
Arteriosclerosis
Diabetes mellitus
Hypertension
Neoplastic angioendotheliosis

Cardiac disease
    Atrial fibrillation
    Congestive heart failure
    Rheumatic heart disease
    Cardiac surgery
    Cardiac myxoma
    Mitral valve prolapse
    Cardiomyopathy
    Prosthetic valve
Inflammatory (non-infectious) vascular disorders
    Systemic lupus erythematosus
    Polyarteritis nodosa
    Rheumatoid arteritis
    Dermatomyositis
    Giant cell arteritis (temporal arteritis)
    Granulomatous arteritis
Chemical causes of vascular disease
    Carbon monoxide poisoning
    Amphetamines
    Ergot derivatives
    Oral contraceptives
Haematological disorders
    Leukaemia
    Lymphoma
    Polycythaemia
    Anaemia
    Hyperlipidaemia
    Disseminated intravascular coagulation
    Cryoglobulinaemia
Metastatic deposits causing vascular obstruction
    Distant malignancy
    Parasites
    Air emboli
    Fat emboli

and inflammatory arteritides and embolic disorders may also produce the syndrome. Table 4.4 presents a classification of common aetiologies of MID.

Treatment. MID is largely irreversible, but early diagnosis and treatment of the underlying condition may prevent further intellectual decline. Treatment should be directed towards lowering elevated blood pressure, preventing further emboli, or prompt treatment of any infectious or haematological disorder. MID is often complicated by depression or psychoses that may respond to antidepressant or antipsychotic treatment.

Binswanger's disease

In 1894, discussing the differential diagnosis of general paresis of the insane, Otto Binswanger described eight cases with progressive dementia, severe atrophy of the white matter and atheromatosis of the arteries of the brain. This disease entity was further described and discussed by Alzheimer, Nissel and Van Bogaert. Olszwesky (1962) was the first to coin the term 'encephalitis subcorticalis chronica progressiva', now known as subcortical arteriosclerotic encephalopathy or Binswanger's disease. Many reports have been published since, and most authors have emphasised the role of vascular disease, the association with hypertension, and the severe atherosclerotic changes of the cerebral arteries and arterioles (Farnell and Globus, 1932). In 1947 Neumann challenged the idea that Binswanger's disease is caused by a vascular process. She suggested that the diseases are found together only coincidentally, and promoted the idea that Binswanger's disease is a demyelinating disorder. Binswanger's disease was then abandoned as a clinical entity for many years. The concept has recently regained popularity with improved technologies that allow its diagnosis in life, and again suggest an intimate relationship with vascular disease.

Clinical characteristics. Binswanger's disease usually presents in the fifth to seventh decades in patients with persistent hypertension and systemic vascular disease. The patient manifests subacute accumulation of focal neurological signs and symptoms, acute strokes, motor signs such as asymmetric weakness with pyramidal signs and pseudobulbar palsy, confusion, gait disturbance and dementia. The disease has a course of three to ten years. During this time periods of stability or even temporary improvement may occur, but the overall course is one of deterioration (Caplan and Schoene, 1978).

Dementia has been reported as a manifestation of the disease since the first description by Binswanger. Patients exhibit psychomotor retardation, have defective judgement, lack spontaneity, manifest long latency when replying to queries, perseverate, lose interest and lack drive (Caplan and Schoene,

1978; Loizou, Kendall and Marshal, 1981). Secondary mania and simple delusions have been reported (Janota, 1981; Jelgersma, 1964; Loizou, *et al.*, 1981). There are also memory impairments, language and speech disturbances, visuospatial difficulties and dilapidation of cognitive functions. The clinical features may be indistinguishable from lacunar state (Rosenberg, Kornfeld, Storring and Bicknell, 1979).

Neuropathology. There is severe cerebral arteriosclerosis and diffuse demyelination of the white matter with ischaemic damage in the deep white matter of the frontal, parietal and occipital lobes. The cerebral cortex and the subcortical arcuate fibres are usually preserved. The basal ganglia, thalami and pontine base typically contain small infarctions (Tomonaga, Yamanouchi, Tohgi and Kameyama, 1982). The long penetrating vessels of the white matter show advanced arteriosclerotic changes. They do not supply the cortex, but course through the cortical mantle and converge near the corner of the lateral ventricles (DeReuck, 1972). These vessels are the same size as

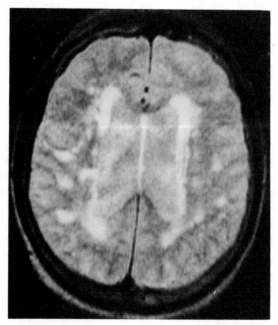

Figure 4.3: Magnetic resonance image (MRI) of a patient with Bingswanger's disease, shows multiple high signal (white) lesions in the white matter of the cerebral hemispheres.

those supplying the basal ganglia, thalami and pons, and are as vulnerable to the development of hypertensive changes in the arterial wall. Dilatation of the ventricles is produced by shrinkage of the periventricular white matter as the disease progresses (Caplan and Schoene, 1978; Kinkel, Lawrence, Polachini, Bates and Heffner, 1985).

Laboratory investigation. Serum and urine studies are unremarkable. CSF is usually normal, although the protein content may be elevated. EEG demonstrates diffuse slowing with minor focal disturbances; periodic complexes have occasionally been reported (Biemond, 1970; White, 1979). CT scan reveals markedly enlarged ventricles with evidence of lacunar infarctions and areas of white matter hypodensity. The latter involve primarily the periventricular white matter and the centrum semiovale. The lesions do not usually enhance with contrast infusion. Magnetic resonance images reveal more pathological lesions than CT scans (Figure 4.3) (Kinkel *et al.,* 1985).

PATHOPHYSIOLOGY OF SUBCORTICAL DEMENTIA

The underlying mechanisms of subcortical dementia remain to be elucidated. However, understanding of the anatomy, pathology, metabolism and neuropsychology of subcortical disorders is improving and the range of functions of the basal ganglia is being revealed. Subcortical structures play a paramount role in mediating, regulating and modulating human behaviour. All diseases reported to produce subcortical dementia routinely involve the striatum (caudate nucleus and putamen) and thalamus with more variable involvement of the substantia nigra, red nucleus, locus coeruleus, subthalamic nucleus, and variably, cerebral cortex (Table 4.2). Atrophy and gliosis of the caudate nucleus is the hallmark pathology in Huntington's disease. In Parkinson's disease the striatum is not structurally affected but because of severe dopamine depletion in the nigrostriatal pathway the striatum is rendered inactive by denervation. In Wilson's disease the pathology affects the lenticular nuclei (putamen and globus pallidus) so severely that they may become cavitated, and in PSP the afferent dopaminergic pathway to the striatum is involved and there is damage to the globus pallidus, subthalamic nuclei and red nuclei. In the spino-cerebellar degenerations the cerebellum and brainstem nuclei are routinely involved with more variable involvement of other components of the basal ganglia.

The basal ganglia are large nuclear masses located subcortically. Nearly all of the neocortex is connected to the basal ganglia by corticofugal fibres originating in the neocortex and distributed directly to the corpus striatum. The striatum can affect the function of the cortex by way of the exit route leading via the pallidum to the thalamic nuclei and then the cerebral cortex. Recently it has become evident that the ventral part of the striatum receives limbic innervation (Nauta and Feirtag, 1986) and shares the same outflow pathway described above, expanding the striatal influence on the neocortex to the limbic system. The outflow tracts for striatal motor and limbic components are distinctive but share the same targets — the subthalamic nucleus and substantia nigra. Thus any pathophysiological process that involves the basal ganglia will affect the motor system, limbic function and subcortical–frontal projections leading to motor disturbances, behaviour alterations and cognitive dysfunction respectively. Table 4.2 summarises the sites of anatomical pathology in common subcortical dementias.

Anatomical pathology, however, is only one means of producing subcortical dysfunction. Disruption of neurotransmitter systems can imitate anatomical damage or can independently produce clinical disturbances (Table 4.3). The principal transmitters implicated in subcortical dementia are dopamine, norepinephrine, GABA and acetylcholine. The occurrence of subcortical dementia in MPTP-induced parkinsonism demonstrates the crucial role of dopamine in intellectual function. MPTP, a synthetic meperidine derivative, produces an essentially pure hypodopaminergic state involving exclusively the nigrostriatal projection (Ballard, Tetrud and Langston, 1985; Davis, Williams, Markey, Ebert, Caine, Reichert and Kopin, 1979; Stern and Langston, 1985). The patients manifest depression, psychomotor retardation, visuospatial disturbances and memory impairment — the principal characteristics of subcortical dementia. These findings suggest that dopamine deficiency may play a critical role in the dementias associated with Parkinson's disease and PSP where dopamine levels are also known to be substantially decreased.

A role for norepinephrine in the manifestations of subcortical dementia was implied by the observation that performance on concentration tasks by patients with Parkinson's disease correlated with CSF levels of 3-methoxy-4-hydroxy-phenylglycol (MHPG), a norepinephrine metabolite (Mayeux, 1984).

GABA and related enzymes are preferentially affected in Huntington's disease, suggesting that this transmitter system also makes essential contributions to human cognition. GABA-ergic and dopaminergic systems have abundant interchanges, and their involvement may have similar effects on mental activity.

The role of acetylcholine loss in subcortical disorders remains to be determined. Cholinergic system enzymes are reduced in most patients with Parkinson's disease with overt dementia (Perry *et al*, 1983). Levels are moderately decreased in some patients with PSP but the reduction correlates poorly with the degree of dementia (Kish, Chong, Mirchandani, Shannak and Hornykiewicz, 1985; Ruberg, Javoy-Agid, Hirsch, Scatton, L'Heurene, Hauw, Duyckaerts, Gray, Morel-Maroger, Rascol, Serdaru and Agid, 1985). In these conditions, acetylcholine deficits may exaggerate symptoms produced by other neurotransmitter abnormalities. Table 4.3 summarises the neurochemical disturbances in subcortical dementia syndromes.

PET and cerebral blood flow techniques have added to understanding of subcortical mechanisms and their influence on behaviour and motility. PET studies in Huntington's disease reveal a distinctive pattern of metabolism characterised by decreased activity of the caudate nuclei and putamen and normal cerebral cortical metabolism (Kuhl, *et al.*, 1982). This contrasts with cortical hypometabolism and relative intact subcortical metabolic activity observed in DAT (Benson *et al.*, 1983) and supports the suggestion that the dementia of HD reflects subcortical dysfunction. PET studies in PSP demonstrate a highly significant hypometabolism in the prefrontal cortex consistent with the suspected impact of PSP on subcortical–frontal projections (D'Anota, Baron, Sanson, Serdaru, Viader, Agid and Canbier, 1985).

In Parkinson's disease, Kuhl, Metter and Riege (1984) found globally decreased brain metabolism. Regional cerebral blood flow was found to be higher in the contralateral cortex in hemi-Parkinson's disease (Wolfson, Leenders, Brown and Jones, 1985). These findings may reflect an abnormality of the dopaminergic innervation of the blood vessels or a true diminished level of metabolic activity. Metabolic studies of other subcortical disorders with dementia are not yet available.

CONCLUSIONS

This review summarises the neuropsychological, neurochemical and neuroanatomical correlates of subcortical dementia, and reviews the principal disorders in which the syndrome occurs. The cardinal neuropsychological characteristics include slowing of mental processes, dilapidation of intellectual cohesion and strategy formation, disruption of recall functions and a variety of personality and mood disturbances. Measurable abnormalities involve reaction times, a variety of continuous performance measures, recent and remote recall, visuospatial abilities, and tasks requiring abstraction, shifting of set and motor programming. Articulation, motor tone, co-ordination and control of adventitious movements are all disturbed.

The principal neurotransmitter involved in the subcortical dementias is dopamine, but roles for norepinephrine, GABA and acetylcholine are suggested by post-mortem neurochemical analyses. Anatomically, the caudate and putamen and their outflow via globus pallidus to thalamic nuclei, and thence to frontal cortex, is the circuit compromised in the subcortical dementias. Influences from involvement of substantia nigra, subthalamic nucleus and ascending brainstem tracts are also likely. The robust afferent and efferent connections between subcortical nuclei and frontal lobes provide an anatomical basis for the clinical similarities between subcortical dementias and frontal lobe syndromes.

Conceptually the subcortical dementia syndrome arises from involvement of fundamental functions such as arousal, timing, mood, motivation, reward and rate of information processing mediated primarily by subcortical structures, whereas the cortical dementia syndrome reflects loss of instrumental functions such as language, praxis and gnosis mediated by the cerebral cortex. Subcortical structures are composed of shorter, less well-myelinated neurones with little lateral specialisation; the cerebral cortex is composed of unique functional units connected by longer, well-myelinated neurones. Lateral specialisation occurs primarily at the cortical level. The two dementia syndromes reflect involvement of two contrasting aspects of

CNS mediation of intellectual activity (Cummings, 1986).

Management of patients is also aided by recognising the cortical or subcortical nature of the dementia syndrome (Shapira, Schlesinger and Cummings, 1986). Patients with subcortical dementia require attention to their movement disorder and usually respond at least partially to pharmacological and physical therapy and social support. When they become slow and depressed a structured environment and an understanding supportive family, along with the proper medical treatment, become crucial. Patients with cortical dementias have no motor disorder throughout most of the clinical course, have no available specific pharmacotherapy, respond poorly to cues, and must be provided with a safe, contained environment.

Thus the two principal patterns of intellectual disturbance reviewed here have contrasting clinical presentations and reflect involvement of different anatomical structures and neurobehavioural mechanisms. Further moulding and differentiation of this nosological approach is likely, but recognition of the two syndromes improves diagnostic accuracy, enhances patient care and expands knowledge of the manner in which intellectual activity is mediated by the nervous system.

ACKNOWLEDGEMENTS

This project was supported by the Veterans Administration. The manuscript was prepared by Norene Hiekel.

REFERENCES

Akelaitis, A.J. (1937–8) Hereditary form of primary parenchymatous atrophy of the cerebellar cortex associated with mental retardation. *American Journal of Psychiatry, 9,* 1115–37

Albert, M.L. Subcortical dementia. (1978) In R. Katzman, R.D. Terry and K.L. Bick (eds), *Alzheimer's disease: senile dementia and related disorders.* Raven Press, New York, pp. 173–80

Albert, M.L., Feldman, R.G. and Willis, A.L. (1974) The 'subcortical dementia' of progressive supranuclear palsy. *Journal of Neurology, Neurosurgery, and Psychiatry, 37,* 121–30

Albert, M.S., Butters, N. and Brandt, J. (1981) Patterns of remote memory in amnestic and demented patients. *Archives of Neurology, 38,* 495–500

Ballard, P.A., Tetrud, J.W. and Langston, J.W. (1985) Permanent

111

human parkinsonism due to 1-methyl-4-phenyl-1,2,3,6-tetrahydro-pyrodine (MPTP): seven cases. *Neurology, 35,* 949–56

Bassi, S., Albizzati, M.G., Corsini, G.U., Frattola, L., Pioleti, R., Suchy, I. and Trabucchi, M. (1986) Therapeutic experience with transhy-drolisuride in Huntington's disease. *Neurology, 36,* 984–6

Beardsley, J.V. and Puletti, F. (1971) Personality (MMPI) and cogni-tive (WAIS) changes after levodopa treatment. *Archives of Neurol-ogy, 25,* 145–50

Beck, J.C., Benson, D.F. and Scheibel, A.B. (1982) Dementia in the elderly: the silent epidemic. *Annals of Internal Medicine, 97,* 231–41

Behrman, C. and Matthews, J. (1969) Progressive supranuclear palsy: clinicopathological study of four cases. *Brain,, 92,* 663–78

Benson, D.F. (1983) Subcortical dementia: a clinical approach. In R.M. Mayeux and W.G. Rosen (eds), *The dementias,* Raven Press, New York, pp. 185–94

Benson, D.F. and Cummings, J.L. (1986) A scheme to differentiate the dementias. In Jeste, D.V. (ed.), *Neuropsychiatric dementias.* Ameri-can Psychiatric Press, Washington, DC, pp. 1–25.

Benson, D.F., Kuhl, D.E., Hawkins, R.A., Phelps, M.E., Cummings, J.L. and Tsai, S.Y. (1983) The fluoro-deoxyglucose ^{18}F scan in Alzheimer's disease and multi-infarct dementia. *Archives of Neurol-ogy, 40,* 711–14

Bentson, T.R. and Keesey, J.C. (1974) Pneumoencephalography in progressive supranuclear palsy. *Radiology, 92,* 89–94

Berciano, J. (1982) Olivopontocerebellar atrophy: a review of 117 cases. *Journal of the Neurological Sciences, 53,* 253–72

Biemond, A. (1970) On Binswanger's subcortical arteriosclerotic encephalopathy and the possibility of its clinical recognition. *Psychi-atria, Neurologia, and Neurochirurgia, 73,* 413–15

Birkett, D.P. and Raskin, A. (1982) Arteriosclerosis, infarcts and dementia. *Journal of the American Geriatric Society, 30,* 261–5

Blumental, H. and Miller, C. (1969) Motor nuclear involvement in progressive supranuclear palsy. *Archives of Neurology, 20,* 362–7

Boll, T.J., Heaton, R. and Reitan, R.M. (1974) Neuropsychological and emotional correlates of Huntington's chorea. *Journal of Nervous and Mental Disease, 158,* 61–9

Boller, F., Mizutani, T., Roesmann, V. and Gambetti, P. (1980) Parkin-son disease, dementia, and Alzheimer disease: clinicopathological correlations. *Annals of Neurology, 7,* 329–35

Boller, F., Passafiume, D., Keefe, N.C., Rogers, K., Morrow, L. and Kim, Y. (1984) Visuospatial impairment in Parkinson's disease: role of perceptual and motor factors. *Archives of Neurology, 41,* 485–94

Bowen, F.P., Kamienny, R.S., Burns, M.M. and Yahr, M.D. (1975) Parkinsonism: effects of levodopa treatment on concept formation. *Neurology, 25,* 701–4

Bromberg, W. (1930) Mental states in chronic encephalitis. *Psychiatric Quarterly, 4,* 537–66

Brouwers, P., Cox, C., Martin, A., Chase, T. and Fedio, P. (1984) Differential perceptual–spatial impairment in Huntington's and

Alzheimer's dementias. *Archives of Neurology, 41*, 1073–6

Brown, G.L. and Wilson, W.P. (1972) Parkinsonism and depression. *Southern Medical Journal, 65*, 540–5

Brown, R.G. and Marsden, C.D. (1984) How common is dementia in Parkinson's disease? *Lancet, 2*, 1262–5

Bulens, C., Meerwaldt, T.D., Van der Wildt, G.J. and Keemink, C.J. (1986) Contrast sensitivity in Parkinson's disease. *Neurology, 36*, 1121–5

Butters, N., Sax, D., Montgomery, K. and Tarlow, S. (1978) Comparison of the neuropsychological deficits associated with early and advanced Huntington's disease. *Archives of Neurology, 35*, 585–9

Caine, E.D. (1981) Pseudodementia; current concepts and future directions. *Archives of General Psychiatry, 38*, 1359–64

Caine, E.D. and Shoulson, I. (1983) Psychiatric syndromes in Huntington's disease. *American Journal of Psychiatry, 140*, 728–33

Caine, E.D., Bamford, K.A., Schiffer, R.B., Shoulson, I. and Levy, S. (1986) A controlled neuropsychological comparison of Huntington's disease and multiple sclerosis. *Archives of Neurology, 43*, 249–54

Caine, E.D., Hunt, R.D., Weingartner, H. and Elbert, M.H. (1978) Huntington's dementia: clinical and neuropsychological features. *Archives of General Psychiatry, 35*, 377–84

Caplan, L.R. (1980) 'Top of the basilar' syndrome. *Neurology, 30*, 72–9

Caplan, L.R. and Schoene, W.C. (1978) Clinical features of subcortical arteriosclerotic encephalopathy (Binswanger disease). *Neurology, 28*, 1206–15

Carter, H.R. and Sukavajuna, C. (1956) Familial cerebello-olivary degeneration with late development of rigidity and dementia. *Neurology, 6*, 876–84

Celesia, G.G and Wannamaker, W.M. (1972) Psychiatric disturbances in Parkinson's disease. *Diseases of the Nervous System, 33*, 577–83

Chandler, J.H. and Bebin, J. (1956) Hereditary cerebellar ataxia: olivopontocerebellar type. *Neurology, 6*, 187–95

Cummings, J.L. (1985) Organic delusions: phenomenology, anatomical correlations, and review. *British Journal of Psychiatry, 146*, 184–97

Cummings, J.L. (1986) Subcortical dementia. *British Journal of Psychiatry, 149*, 682–97

Cummings, J.L. and Benson, D.F. (1983) *Dementia: a clinical approach.* Butterworths, Boston

Cummings, J.L. and Benson, D.F. (1986) Dementia of the Alzheimer's type: an inventory of diagnostic clinical features. *Journal of the American Geriatrics Society, 34*, 12–19

Cummings, J.L. and Mendez, M.F. (1984) Secondary mania with focal cerebrovascular lesions. *American Journal of Psychiatry, 141*, 1084–91

Cummings, J.L., Benson, D.F., Houlihan, J.P. and Gosenfeld, L.F. (1983a) Mutism: loss of neocortical and limbic vocalization. *Journal of Nervous and Mental Disease, 171*, 255–9

Cummings, J.L., Gosenfeld, L., Houlihan, J. and McCaffrey, T. (1983b) Neuropsychiatric manifestations of idiopathic calcification

113

of the basal ganglia: case report and review. *Biological Psychiatry, 18,* 591–601

Danta, G. and Hilton, R.C. (1975) Judgement of the visual vertical and horizontal in patients with parkinsonism. *Neurology, 25,* 43–7

D'Antona, R., Baron, J.C., Sanson, Y., Serdaru, M., Viader, F., Agid, Y. and Canbier, J. (1985) Subcortical dementia; frontal cortex hypometabolism detected by positron tomography in patients with progressive supranuclear palsy. *Brain, 108,* 785–99

Davies, D.L. (1949) Intelligence of patients with Friedreich's ataxia. *Journal of Neurology, Neurosurgery and Psychiatry, 12,* 34–8, 246–50

Davis, G.C., Williams, A.C., Markey, S.P., Ebert, M.H., Caine, E.D., Reichert, C.M. and Kopin, I.J. (1979) Chronic parkinsonism secondary to intravenous injection of mepiridine analogues. *Psychiatry Research, 1,* 249–54

Davis, P.H., Bergerow, C. and McLachlan, D.R. (1985) Atypical presentation of progressive supranuclear palsy. *Annals of Neurology, 17,* 337–43

Denny-Brown, D. (1964) Hepatolenticular degeneration (Wilson's disease). *New England Journal of Medicine, 270,* 1149–56

DeReuck, J.D. (1972) The cortico-subcortical arterial angio-architecture in the human brain. *Acta Neurologica Belgica, 72,* 323–9

Dewhurst, K., Oliver, J.E. and McKnight, A.L. (1970) Socio-psychiatric consequences of Huntington's disease. *British Journal of Psychiatry, 116,* 255–8

Direnfeld, L.K., Albert, M.L., Volicer, L., Langlais, P.J., Marquis, J. and Kaplan, E. (1984) Parkinson's disease: the possible relationship of laterality to dementia and neurochemical findings. *Archives of Neurology, 41,* 935–41

Evarts, E.V., Teravainen, H. and Calne, D.B. (1981) Reaction time in Parkinson's disease. *Brain, 104,* 167–86

Fairweather, D.S. (1947) Psychiatric aspects of the post-encephalitic syndrome. *Journal of Mental Science, 93,* 201–54

Farnell, F.J. and Globus, T.H. (1932) Chronic progressive vascular subcortical encephalopathy. *Archives of Neurology and Psychiatry, 27,* 593–604

Fields, W.S. (1986) Multi-infarct dementia. *Neurologic Clinics, 4,* 405–13

Fisk, J.D., Goodale, M.A., Burkhart, G. and Barnett, H.T.M. (1982) Progressive supranuclear palsy: the relationship between ocular motor dysfunction and psychological test performance. *Neurology, 32,* 698–705

Folstein, S.E., Franz, M.L., Jensen, B.A., Chase, G.A. and Folstein, M.F. (1983) Conduct disorder and affective disorder among the offspring of patients with Huntington disease. *Psychological Medicine, 13,* 45–52

Freedman, M., Rivoria, P., Butters, N., Sax, D.S. and Feldman, R.G. (1984) Retrograde amnesia in Parkinson's disease. *Canadian Journal of Neurological Science, 11,* 297–301

Girrotti, F., Carella, F., Grassi, M.P., Soliveri, P., Marano, R. and

Caraceni, T. (1986) Motor and cognitive performance of parkinsonian patients in the on and off phase of the disease. *Journal of Neurology, Neurosurgery, and Psychiatry*, 49, 657–60

Goldstein, N.P., Ewart, J.C., Randall, R.V. and Gross, J.B. (1968) Psychiatric aspects of Wilson's disease (hepatolenticular degeneration): result of psychometric tests during long term therapy. *American Journal of Psychiatry*, *124*, 1555–61

Greenfield, J.G. (1954) *The spinocerebellar degenerations.* Blackwell Scientific Publications, Oxford

Greenfield, J.G. and Bosanquet, F.D. (1953) The brain-stem lesions in parkinsonism. *Journal of Neurology, Neurosurgery, and Psychiatry*, *16*, 213–26

Hachinski, V.C. (1983) Multi-infarct dementia. *Neurologic Clinics, 1*, 27–36

Hachinski, V.C., Iliff, L.D., Zilhka, E., Du Boulay, G., McAllister, V.L., Marshall, J., Russell, R.W.R. and Symon, L. (1975) Cerebral blood flow in dementia. *Archives of Neurology, 32*, 632–7

Hachinski, V.C., Lassen, N.A. and Marshall, J. (1974) Multi-infarct dementia: a cause of mental deterioration in the elderly. *Lancet, 2*, 207–10

Hakim, A.M. and Mathieson, G. (1979) Dementia in Parkinson disease: a neuropathologic study. *Neurology, 29*, 1209–14

Haldeman, S., Goldman, J.W., Hyde, J. and Pribram, H.F. (1981) Progressive supranuclear palsy, computed tomography and response to anti-parkinsonian drugs. *Neurology, 3*, 442–5

Halgin, R., Riklan, M. and Misiak, H. (1977) Levodopa, parkinsonism, and recent memory. *Journal of Nervous and Mental Disease, 164*, 268–72

Hamilton, N.G., Frick, R.B., Takahashi, T. and Hopping, M.W. (1983) Psychiatric symptoms and cerebellar pathology. *American Journal of Psychiatry, 140*, 1322–6

Hart, R.P., Kwentus, J.A., Leshner, R.T. and Frazier, R. (1985) Information processing speed in Friedreich's ataxia. *Annals of Neurology, 17*, 612–14

Hayden, M.R. (1981) *Huntington's chorea.* Springer-Verlag, New York

Heston, L.L. (1980) Dementia associated with Parkinson's disease: a genetic study. *Journal of Neurology, Neurosurgery, and Psychiatry, 43*, 846–8

Hecaen, H. and Albert, M.L. (1978) *Human neuropsychology.* Wiley Interscience Publications, New York

Hoehn, M.M., Crowley, T.J. and Rutledge, C.O. (1976) Dopamine correlates of neurological and psychological status in untreated parkinsonism. *Journal of Neurology, Neurosurgery, and Psychiatry, 39*, 941–51

Hornykiewicz, O. (1973) Parkinson's disease: from brain homogenate to treatment. *Federation Proceedings, 32*, 183–90

Ishino, H., Higashi, H., Kuroda, S., Yabuki, S., Hayahara, T. and Otsuki, S. (1974) Motor nuclear involvement in progressive supranuclear palsy. *Journal of the Neurological Sciences, 22*, 235–44

Jackson, J.A., Jankovic, J. and Ford, J. (1983) Progressive supranuclear palsy: clinical features and response treatment in 16 patients. *Annals of Neurology*, *13*, 273–8

Jankovic, J. (1984) Progressive supranuclear palsy: clinical and pharmacological update. *Neurologic Clinics*, *2*, 473–86

Janota, I. (1981) Dementia, deep white matter damage and hypertension. 'Binswanger's disease'. *Psychological Medicine*, *11*, 39–48

Javoy-Agid, F. and Agid, Y. (1980) Is the mesocortical dopaminergic system involved in Parkinson disease? *Neurology*, *30*, 1326–30

Jelgersma, H.C. (1964) A case of encephalopathia subcorticalis chronica (Binswanger's disease). *Psychiatrica et Neurologica (Basel)*, *147*, 81–9

Jellinger, K. (1976) Neuropathological aspects of dementia resulting from abnormal blood flow and cerebrospinal fluid dynamics. *Acta Neurologica Belgica*, *76*, 83–102

Kark, R.A.P. and Rodriquez-Budelli, M.M. (1979) Clinical correlations of lipoamide dehydrogenase. *Neurology*, *29*, 1006–13

Kase, C.S. (1986) 'Multi-infarct' dementia: a real entity? *Journal of the American Geriatrics Society*, *34*, 482–4

Kiloh, L.G., McComas, A.J. and Osselton, J.W. (1972) *Clinical electroencephalography*, 3rd edn. Butterworths, London

Kimura, D., Barnett, H.J.M. and Burkhart, G. (1981) The psychological test pattern in progressive supranuclear palsy. *Neuropsychologia*, *19*, 301–6

Kinkel, W.R., Lawrence, J., Polachini, I., Bates, V. and Heffner, R.R. (1985) Subcortical arteriosclerotic encephalopathy (Binswanger's disease). *Archives of Neurology*, *42*, 951–9

Kish, S.J., Chong, L.J., Mirchandani, L., Shannak, K. and Hornykiewicz, O. (1985) Progressive supranuclear palsy: relationship between extrapyramidal disturbances, dementia, and brain neurotransmitter markers. *Annals of Neurology*, *18*, 530–6

Klawans, H.L. Jr and Ringel, S.P. (1971) Observation of the efficacy of levodopa in progressive supranuclear palsy. *European Neurology*, *5*, 115–29

Knehr, C.A. and Bearn, A.G. (1956) Psychological impairment in Wilson's disease. *Journal of Nervous and Mental Disease*, *124*, 251–5

Kuhl, D.E., Metter, E.J. and Riege, W.H. (1984) Patterns of local cerebral glucose utilization determined in Parkinson's disease by the [18F] fluorodeoxyglucose method. *Annals of Neurology*, *15*, 419–24

Kuhl, D.E., Phelps, M.E., Markham, C.H., Metter, E.J., Riege, W.H. and Winter, J. (1982) Cerebral metabolism and atrophy in Huntington's disease determined by 18F-DG and computed tomographic scan. *Annals of Neurology*, *12*, 425–34

Lance, J.W., Schwab, R.S. and Peterson, E.R. (1963) Action tremor and the cogwheel phenomenon in Parkinson's disease. *Brain*, *86*, 95–109

Lees, A.J. and Smith, E. (1983) Cognitive deficits in the early stages of Parkinson's disease. *Brain*, *106*, 257–70

Lieberman, A., Dziatolowski, M., Kupersmith, M., Serby, M., Goodgold, A., Korein, J. and Goldstein, M. (1979) Dementia in Parkinson disease. *Annals of Neurology*, 6, 355–9

Loizou, L.A., Kendall, B.E. and Marshal, J. (1981) Subcortical arteriosclerotic encephalopathy: a clinical and radiological investigation. *Journal of Neurology, Neurosurgery and Psychiatry*, 44, 294–304

Loranger, A.W., Goodell, H., McDowell, F.H., Lee, J.E. and Sweet, R.D. (1972) Intellectual impairment in Parkinson's syndrome. *Brain*, 95, 405–12

Maher, E.R., Smith, E.M. and Lees, A.J. (1985) Cognitive deficits in Steele–Richardson–Olszewski syndrome (progressive supranuclear palsy). *Journal of Neurology, Neurosurgery and Psychiatry*, 48, 1234–9

Martone, M., Butters, N., Payne, M., Becker, J.T. and Sax, D.S. (1984) Dissociation between skill learning and verbal recognition in amnesia and dementia. *Archives of Neurology*, 41, 965–70

Mastaglia, F.L., Grainger, K.G., Kee, F., Sadk, A.M. and Lefroy, R. (1973) Progressive supranuclear palsy (the Steele–Richardson–Olszewski syndrome): clinical and electrophysiological observations in eleven patients. *Proceedings of the Australian Association of Neurology*, 10, 35–44

Mayeux, R. (1984) Behavioral manifestation of movement disorders: Parkinson's and Huntington's disease. *Neurologic Clinics*, 2, 527–40

McDowell, F.H., Lee, J.E. and Sweet, R.D. (1978) Extrapyramidal disease. In A.B. Baker and R.J. Joynt (eds), *Clinical neurology*. Harper & Row, New York, pp. 1–67

McHugh, P.R. and Folstein, M.F. (1975) Psychiatric syndromes of Huntington's chorea: a clinical and phenomenologic study. In D.F. Benson and D. Blumer (eds), *Psychiatric aspects of neurologic disease*. Grune & Stratton, New York, pp. 267–85

Meier, M.J. and Martin, W.E. (1970) Intellectual changes associated with levodopa therapy. *Journal of the American Medical Association*, 213, 465–6

Mesulam, M.M. (1985) Attention, confusional states and neglect. In M.M. Mesulam (ed.), *Principles of behavioral neurology*. F.A. Davis, Philadelphia, pp. 125–68

Moss, M.B., Albert, M.S., Butters, N. and Payne, M. (1986) Differential patterns of memory loss among patients with Alzheimer's disease, Huntington's disease, and alcoholic Korsakoff's syndrome. *Archives of Neurology*, 43, 239–46

Nauta, W.J.H. and Feirtag, M. (1986) *Fundamental neuroanatomy*. W.H. Freeman, New York

Nelson, R.F., Guzman, D.A., Grahovac, Z. and Howse, C.D.N. (1979) Computerized cranial tomography in Wilson's disease. *Neurology*, 29, 866–8

Neophytides, A., Liberman, A.N., Goldstein, M., Gopinathan, G., Leibowitz, M., Bock, J. and Walker, R. (1982) The use of lisuride, a potent dopamine and serotonin agonist, in the treatment of progressive supranuclear palsy. *Journal of Neurology, Neurosurgery and Psychiatry*, 45, 261–3

Netsky, M.G. (1968) Degeneration of the cerebellum and its pathways. In J. Minckler (ed.), *Pathology of the nervous system*. McGraw-Hill, New York, pp. 1163–85

Neumann, M.A. (1947) Chronic progressive subcortical encephalopathy: report of a case. *Journal of Gerontology*, 2, 57–64

Newman, G.C. (1985) Treatment of progressive supranuclear palsy with tricyclic antidepressants. *Neurology*, 35, 1189–93

Obler, L.K., Cummings, M.L. and Albert, M.L. (1979) Subcortical dementia: speech and language functions. Paper presented at the American Geriatric Society Meeting, Washington, DC, April

Olszewsky, J. (1962) Subcortical arteriosclerotic encephalopathy. *World Neurology*, 3, 359–75

Oppenheimer, D.R. (1976) Diseases of the basal ganglia, cerebellum, and motor neurons. In W. Blackwood and J.A.N. Corsellis (eds), *Greenfield's neuropathology*. Yearbook Medical Publishers, Chicago, pp. 608–51

Parkes, J.D., Baxter, R.C.H., Curson, G., Knill-Jones, R.P., Knott, P.J., Marsden, C.D., Tattersall, R. and Vellum, D. (1971) Treatment of Parkinson's disease with amantadine and levodopa. *Lancet*, i, 1083–6

Parkinson, J. (1817) *An essay on the shaking palsy*. Sherwood, Neely & Jones, London

Perry, E.K., Perry, R.N., Blessed, G. and Tomlinson, B.E. (1977) Necropsy evidence of central cholinergic deficits in senile dementia. *Lancet*, i, 189

Perry, R.H., Tomlinson, B.E., Candy, J.M., Blessed, G., Foster, J.F., Bloxham, C.A. and Perry, E.R. (1983) Cortical cholinergic deficit in mentally impaired parkinsonian patients. *Lancet*, ii, 789–90

Pillon, B., Dubois, B., Lermitte, F. and Agid, Y. (1986) Heterogeneity of cognitive impairment in progressive supranuclear palsy, Parkinson's disease, and Alzheimer's disease. *Neurology*, 36, 1179–85

Pincus, J.H. and Tucker, G.J. (1985) *Behavioral neurology*. Oxford University Press, New York

Pirozzolo, F.J., Hansch, E.C., Mortimer, J.A., Webster, D.A. and Kuskowski, M.A. (1982) Dementia in Parkinson's disease: a neuropsychological analysis. *Brain and Cognition*, 1, 71–83

Plum, F. and Posner, J.B. (1980) *The diagnosis of stupor and coma*, 3rd edn. F.A. Davis, Philadelphia

Pollock, M. and Hornabrook, R.W. (1966) The prevalence, natural history and dementia of Parkinson's disease. *Brain*, 89, 429–88

Powell, H.C., London, G.W. and Lampert, P.W. (1974) Neurofibrillary tangles in progressive supranuclear palsy. *Journal of Neuropathology and Experimental Neurology*, 33, 98–106

Proctor, F., Riklan, M., Cooper, I.S. and Teuber, H.L. (1964) Judgement of visual and vertical by parkinsonian patients. *Neurology*, 14, 287–93

Rafal, R.D. and Grimm, R.J. (1981) Progressive supranuclear palsy: functional analysis of the response to methysergide and antiparkinsonian agents. *Neurology*, 31, 1507–18

Reitan, R.M. and Boll, T.J. (1971) Intellectual and cognitive functioning in Parkinson's disease. *Journal of Consulting and Clinical Psychology, 37,* 364–9

Rekate, H.L., Grubb, R.L., Aram, D.M., Hahn, J.F. and Ratcheson, R.A. (1985) Muteness of cerebellar origin. *Archives of Neurology, 42,* 697–8

Rosenbaum, D. (1941) Psychosis with Huntington's disease. *Psychiatric Quarterly, 15,* 93–9

Rosenberg, G.A., Kornfeld, M., Storring, J. and Bicknell, J.M. (1979) Subcortical arteriosclerotic encephalopathy (Binswanger): computerized tomography. *Neurology, 29,* 1102–6

Roy, S., Datta, C.K., Hirano, A., Ghatak, N.R. and Zimmerman, H.M. (1974) Electron microscopic study of neurofibrillary tangles in Steele–Richardson–Olszewski syndrome. *Acta Neuropathologica (Berlin), 29,* 175–9

Ruberg, M., Javoy-Agid, F., Hirsch, E., Scatton, B., L'Heurene, R., Hauw, J.-J., Duyckaerts, C., Gray, F., Morel-Maroger, A., Rascol, A., Serdaru, M. and Agid, Y. (1985) Dopaminergic and cholinergic lesions in progressive supranuclear palsy. *Annals of Neurology, 18,* 523–9

Sacks, O.W., Kohl, M.S., Messeloff, C.R. and Schwartz, W.F. (1972) Effects of levodopa in parkinsonian patients with dementia. *Neurology, 27,* 516–19

Schoenfeld, M., Myers, R.H., Cupples, L.A., Berkman, B., Sax, D.S. and Clark, E. (1984) Increased rate of suicide among patients with Huntington's disease. *Journal of Neurology, Neurosurgery, and Psychiatry, 47,* 1283–7

Shapira, J., Schlesinger, R. and Cummings, J.L. (1986) Distinguishing dementias. *American Journal of Nursing, 54,* 698–702

Shepherd, M. (1955) Report of a family suffering from Friedreich's disease, peroneal muscular atrophy and schizophrenia. *Journal of Neurology, Neurosurgery, and Psychiatry, 18,* 297–304

Shoulson, I. (1981) Functional capacities in patients treated with neuroleptics and antidepressant drugs. *Neurology, 31,* 1333–5

Shoulson, I. (1984) Huntington's disease: a decade of progress. *Neurologic Clinics, 2,* 515–25

Shults, C., Steardo, L., Barone, P., Mohr, E., Juncos, J., Serrati, C., Fedio, P., Tammingo, C.A. and Chase, T.M. (1986) Huntington's disease: effect of cysteamine, a somatostatin depleting agent. *Neurology, 36,* 1099–1102

Steele, J.C. (1972) Progressive supranuclear palsy. *Brain, 95,* 693–704

Steele, J.C., Richardson, J.C. and Olszewski, J. (1964) Progressive supranuclear palsy. *Archives of Neurology, 10,* 333–59

Stern, Y. and Langston, J.W. (1985) Intellectual changes in patients with MPTP-induced parkinsonism. *Neurology, 35,* 1506–9

Stone, T.T. and Folstein, E.I. (1939) Genealogical studies in Huntington's chorea. *Journal of Nervous and Mental Disease, 89,* 795–809

Tanahashi, N., Meyer, J.S., Ishikawa, Y., Kandula, P., Morte, K.F., Rogers, R.L., Gandhi, S. and Walker, M. (1985) Cerebral blood flow and cognitive testing correlate in Huntington's disease. *Archives of Neurology, 42,* 1169–75

Tellez–Nagel, I. and Wisniewski, H.M. (1973) Ultrastructure of neuro-fibrillary tangles in Steele–Richardson–Olszewski syndrome. *Archives of Neurology, 29,* 324–7

Tomlinson, B.E., Blessed, G. and Roth, M. (1970) Observations on the brains of demented old people. *Journal of the Neurological Sciences, 11,* 205–42

Tomonaga, M. (1977) Ultrastructure of neurofibrillary tangles in progressive supranuclear palsy. *Acta Neuropathologica (Berlin), 37,* 177–89

Tomonaga, M., Yamanouchi, H., Tohgi, H. and Kameyama, M. (1982) Clinico-pathologic study of progressive subcortical vascular encephalopathy (Binswanger type) in the elderly. *Journal of the American Geriatrics Society, 30,* 524–9

Trimble, M.R. and Cummings, J.L. (1981) Neuropsychiatric disturbances following brain stem lesions. *British Journal of Psychiatry, 138,* 56–9

Troost, B.T. and Daroff, R.B. (1977) The ocular motor defects in progressive supranuclear palsy. *Annals of Neurology, 2,* 397–403

Uhl, G.R., Hackney, G.O., Torchia, M., Stranov, V., Tourtellotte, W.W., Whitehouse, P.J., Tran, V. and Strittmatter, S. (1986) Parkinson's disease: nigral receptor changes support peptidergic role in nigrostriatal modulation. *Annals of Neurology, 20,* 194–203

Villardita, C., Smirni, P. and Zappala, G. (1983) Visual neglect in Parkinson's disease. *Archives of Neurology, 40,* 737–9

White, J.C. (1979) Periodic EEG activity in subcortical arteriosclerotic encephalopathy (Binswanger's type). *Archives of Neurology, 36,* 485–9

Whitehouse, P.J., Hedreen, J.C., White, C.L. III and Price, D.L. (1983) Basal forebrain neurons in the dementia of Parkinson's disease. *Annals of Neurology, 13,* 243–8

Whittier, J., Haydn, G. and Crawford, J. (1961) Effect of imipramine (Tofranil) on depression and hyperkinesia in Huntington's disease. *American Journal of Psychiatry, 118,* 79

Wikkelso, C., Blomstrand, C. and Nordoquist, P. (1981) Cerebrospinal fluid investigations in multi-infarct dementia and senile dementia. *Acta Neurologica Scandinavia, 64,* 1–11

Wilson, S.A.K. (1912) Progressive lenticular degeneration: a familial nervous disease associated with cirrhosis of the liver. *Brain, 34,* 295–509

Wilson, R.S., Kaszniak, H.L., Klawans, H.L. and Garron, D.C. (1980) High speed memory scanning in parkinsonism. *Cortex, 16,* 67–72

Wolfson, L.J., Leenders, K.L., Brown, L.L. and Jones, T. (1985) Alteration of regional cerebral blood flow and oxygen metabolism in Parkinson's disease. *Neurology, 35,* 1399–1405

5

Communication Changes in Normal and Abnormal Ageing

Ian M Thompson

It is estimated that the prevalence of hearing impairments in the aged is 23 per cent in the sixth decade and 40 per cent in the seventh. It is also estimated that up to 25 per cent of patients admitted to geriatric wards are speech or language impaired. In the community about 14 per cent of the normal, healthy elderly produce neurolinguistic errors that place them within dementing range. In spite of these alarming figures disorders of communication in normal ageing and neuropsychiatry are under-researched. The reason is that those who deal with the problem, speech and language pathologists, are not resourced to analyse the clinical data that pack their files.

Increasingly sophisticated language assessments and advances in neurological imaging techniques have made it possible to understand the relationship between linguistic functioning and brain physiology. This marriage of dynamic imaging and cognitive processes has fostered the infant science of neurolinguistics, broadly defined as the study of brain correlates to language. Hitherto normal and abnormal language function has been investigated following diseases of neoplastic and vascular origin, the effects of missile wounds, electrical stimulation of the cortex and computerised tomography. *In vivo* studies of cerebral blood flow and positron emission tomography have imaged the working brain in language functioning. The effects of diffuse and focal brain lesions on 'intelligence' are still disputed. Jackson's comment that 'to localise the damage which destroys speech and to localise speech are two different things' is less true today than it was 100 years ago.

The 'localisationist' school, following phrenology, considered specific areas of the brain were responsible for discrete mental functions. Broca in 1861 demonstrated that speech could be localised in the inferior portion of the third frontal gyrus. Wernicke, in 1874, described two types of aphasia, motor and sensory which were separable. He localised sensory aphasia to the posterior third of the upper temporal convolution. In 1881 Exner suggested a writing centre in the second frontal convolution adjacent to the hand area of the precentral motor strip. Pick, in his paper 'On the relation between aphasia and senile atrophy of the brain', of 1892 emphasised the language of his patients in terms of localisationist classifications of aphasia.

Opposing this position the 'holists' argued that brain functions were equipotential and determined by mass action. Their position was stated by Marie in 1906 and clinically demonstrated in animals by Lashley in 1926. It has been supported by American aphasiologists and German and English neurologists.

In 1965 Geschwind published his 'Disconnection syndromes in animals and man' and revived interest in the localisationist–connectionist model of cerebral functioning. He argued cortical tissue is divided into specific areas of functional importance and linked by complex networks of association fibres. Alexander Luria, the great Russian neuropsychologist, while expressing strong antilocalisationist opinions, argued the brain acts in complex functional dynamic systems of primary, secondary and tertiary zones each differentiated by cytoarchitecture. Cerebral blood flow studies have supported this dynamic concept of cortical functioning in language. There is a continued dispute about the nature of tertiary zones of cross-modal functioning that programme language; however positron tomography has established a dynamic theory of language function related to the theory of metabolic function which makes Luria's concept of interactive neuropsychological interpretations of language and aphasia assume greater significance.

Communication is the major achievement of cognition. It is more than the ability to verbalise; it is the complex synergy of voice, speech, language and paralanguage, and this model provides a hierarchy for an overview of cognitive performance in both normal and abnormal ageing. Voicing demands acoustic and supraglottic features of frequency, intensity and rhythm. Speech involves articulation and prosodic realisation of this acoustic energy while language is the symbolic formulation of linguistic and paralinguistic phenomena.

VOICE

Voice is the acoustic transformation of breath support into energy that is shaped by glottic and supraglottic structures into pitch, loudness and intonation. Dysphonia following senile changes to the larynx has been documented, but there is no evidence of dysphonia in degenerative dementia, although the possibility of aphonia in frontal lobe disease has been raised by Sapir and Aronson (1985).

The fundamental frequency of the voice increases from the fifth to the eighth decades with an accompanying increase of variability and phonation time ratios in men rather than women. There are changes of resonance and loudness with advancing age. Loss of volume relates to diminished ventilatory capacity and the increased susceptibility of the elderly to respiratory disease and osteoporosis, which affect breath support and underpin vocal quality. At laryngeal level increased fundamental frequency of the voice in the aged male may relate to vocal fold atrophy, and breathiness to vocal cord bowing. Thus there is histological evidence and evidence of tension changes in laryngeal speech musculature that appears to account for the characteristic thin, piping and shrill voice one remembers from Shakespeare's penultimate stage in man's progress:

> ... and his big manly voice
> Turning again towards childish treble, pipes
> And whistles in his sound.

Voice disorders in the elderly may result from lifetime abuse. They can be psychological, mechanical or organic in aetiology. The human voice reflects personality and is used as an instrument of persuasion and deceit. Film sirens developed voices that were breathy and with lowered pitch, and contemporary politicians' manufactured voices are strong and strident (even hectoring) on political platforms but breathy and reduced in pitch to convey care, concern and intimacy in interview. Faded news clips of Nazi rallies of the pre-war era demonstrate the brutal shouting voices of unbridled political power vested in thugs. The voices of the stage project personalities; the cold, brittle, harsh voice of Burton and the mellifluence of the urbane Gielgud.

The voice also reflects emotional state as in stage fright,

terror, hysteria, dumbfoundedness and sexual identification.

Poor vocal hygiene and mechanical abuse of the larynx produced dysphonia in singers, schoolboys, auctioneers, teachers and businessmen who force their voices to maintain volume. The larynx is a delicate instrument that sits in the muscle sling. It is not bone but soft pliable cartilage bound by ligaments. Its purpose is to protect the airway and, by valving, to increase interthoracic pressure in effortful work. It has been adapted to facilitate voice by transforming breath support into acoustic energy. External pressures change voice quality, as for example increased musculoskeletal pressure of neck and shoulder strain. Vocal change can be volitional. We can change the adductive ability of the vocal folds into a whisper or flood glottis to mask breathiness. We can alter marginal tension in the vocal cords to sound creaky or vibrate segments of the folds to produce falsetto. The elderly who have distorted their postures throughout their working life at board tables and desks; who have shouted over smoke-filled bars, conference rooms or chalky, dusty atmospheres; or who have paid little attention to their working posture, are at risk of developing a 'geriatric voice syndrome' which is faltering, breathless, unsteady and of diminished volume. Those who have abused their voice with continual tobacco smoking over extended periods are vulnerable to carcinoma of the larynx, and in acute stages those who abuse their voices mechanically are vulnerable to nodules and watery polyps.

Ageing, then, and a lifetime of vocal abuse, produce alterations to the delicate structure of the larynx. This brings myasthenia, weakening of tension of the vocal ligaments and reduced articulation of the laryngeal joints. Vocal mucosa dehydrates, muscle loses elasticity, cartilage calcifies and the vocal cords bow and become flaccid. Postural changes as a characteristic 'dowager's hump' positions the laryngeal set to shoulder level and postural droop decreases the ventilatory capacity of the lungs which provide the reservoir of air for the larynx to transform, and which determines pressures to assist vocal cord adduction.

SPEECH

The lungs are a reservoir for the larynx to transform breath support into acoustic energy, but the vocal tract shapes this energy and realises it as speech. Vowels are determined by tongue height and mobility, and consonants by the shifting and shaping of the articulators, the tongue, palate, teeth and buccal mucosa. Disorders of speech are dysarthrias and are neuromuscular in origin. Speech disturbance may reflect disease of the basal ganglia, cerebellum, the upper and/or lower motor neurone system. There is often an overlap of disorders of voice and speech; the speech of Parkinson's disease is often labelled a dysarthrophonia.

Specific dysarthrias are neurologically described. Lesions to the cranial nerves subserving tongue movement, jaw excursion, the soft palate and the vocal cords produce characteristic patterns. Flaccid dysarthria in Bell's palsy is accompanied by drooling. Spastic dysarthria affecting the vocal cords may produce a strange strangled quality as subglottic pressure cannot overcome laryngeal tension. Bilateral lesions in pseudobulbar palsy produce characteristic raised tension, pitch and breathiness accompanied by changes in emotional control. The speech of Parkinsonism is affected by laryngeal valving with repetitious dysfluency of reduced volume and increased breathiness. There is limited excursion of the articulators, adynamism of patterning, and palilalia, the dysfluent repetition to inaudibility.

In the normal elderly, speech rates as a feature of neuromuscular function diminish. Speed and accuracy of articulation are also diminished beyond the sixth decade and sensory feedback is reduced. There is increased dysfluency which may indicate an increasing search with a rise of articulatory programming. Although dysarthria is by no means common in ageing, the elderly as a group may be at the mild end of a continuum. Ventilatory capacity decreases with age, affecting loudness, and laryngeal changes alter phonation. Alteration of velopharyngeal mechanisms produces a perceptual rise of nasal resonance, and ageing restriction of the temporomandibular joint may alter oral resonance. Speech changes can also be caused by toothlessness, ill-fitting dentures and a loss of muscle bulk from the cheeks which keeps dental plates firm. The net effect is subtle changes to the respiratory, phonatory, articulatory, resonating and prosodic systems. Motor speed, excursion and precision decreases while pausological phenomena make speech more dysfluent.

The elderly have difficulty perceiving speech when it is

temporally extended or compressed. They are poor at comprehending auditory information by rate and complexity. Such disabilities may be related to presbycusis, attention, ambiguity and inflexibility.

Dysarthria in dementia of Alzheimer type has been reported at a rate of 10–30 per cent; however, dysarthria in dementia is secondary to cerebrovascular disease and the subcortical degenerative diseases rather than parenchymal disorders.

LANGUAGE

If, broadly, speech is the way we say something, language is what it is we wish to say or perceive others to say. It is the transforming of our needs and thoughts into verbal symbols. Measurement of language changes in the normal elderly are rare, and a search of the literature of language in normal senescence and early dementia uncovers only occasional case reports and even less frequent attempts at systematic investigation. It is not clear which changes in ageing are normal and which are not.

Elderly people are more susceptible to injury-related changes of language. 80–90 per cent of CNS injuries after the age of 50 are due to stroke, and 70 per cent of strokes occur after the age of 70. The posterior cortex is more vulnerable to age-related strokes producing more fluent Wernicke-type aphasias, and although capacity for improvement of language may be inversely related to age, it may not be the sole predictor of language recovery.

Probably the most dramatic language disorders follow focal lesions to the left hemisphere, which is usually dominant for language in right-handers and 60 per cent of left-handers as well. Such disorders of language are called aphasias. Focal lesions producing aphasic syndromes, or clusters of symptoms, have taught us more about how language is represented in the brain. A classification of aphasias is given in Table 5.1. Lesions to the lateral frontal lobes produce an adynamia of language, lesions to Broca's area produce dysfluent telegraphic language, lesions across the sensory motor strip produce articulatory apraxias. Posterior lesions of the temporal lobe produce comprehension disorders through a failure to decode speech sounds, and lesions to the parietal lobe produce a failure to decode grammatical concepts. Expressively, parietal lesions

Table 5.1: A classification of aphasic syndromes with symptoms

Name of aphasia	Site of lesion	
Sensory (Wernicke's) aphasia	Posterior third superior temporal gyrus	Cannot distinguish, isolate, identify or repeat phonemes. Cannot understand speech, show jargon, automatisms. Cannot name objects. Cannot read or recognise letters. Can copy but not write spontaneously. Retain functions of visual perception, prosody, logicogrammatical relationships, ability to calculate. Cannot be helped by prompting of the first sound or syllable. Reduced awareness of errors.
Acoustic–amnestic aphasia	Inferior temporal lobe	Phonemic hearing only slightly disturbed but audioverbal memory damaged. Cannot retain series of sounds, syllables, words. Can produce short series of successive stimuli given after interval. Tends to give last given stimulus. Cannot recall words. Frequently can write series.
Semantic (nominal) aphasia	Posterior parietal–occipital lobe	Cannot name objects; have less difficulty with adjectives and verbs. Cannot recall clear visual idea of the object required to name. Responds immediately to initial sound or syllable cue. Frequently confuses words belonging to same semantic category. Paraphasia occurs. Can understand individual words, but disturbance in logicogrammatical relationship in language. Inability to see parts in relation to whole. Disturbances in spatial and temporal relations; cannot calculate. Difficulty in drawing letters. Difficulty in finding direction in space. Intonation and melodic structure of sentence retained.
Articulatory dyspraxia	Left central region	Cannot assume correct tongue, lip, etc., position due to

		difficulty in finding particular articuleme. Difficulty in reading aloud and in writing. Substitutions are made between phonemes that are similar in place and manner of production, t/d, l/r, p/m/b.
Motor (Broca's) aphasia	Left premotor area	Cannot move from one sound to another in a word. Speech loses automatic fluency and becomes fragmented and tense. Telegraphic speech may develop with recovery. Melodic structure of speech may be disturbed. Difficulty in transition is complicated by lack of inhibition and preservation. Writing reflects speech pattern: perseveration of a word once written.
Dynamic aphasia	Left inferior pre-frontal region	Cannot initiate and sustain a long passage of speech (spontaneous). Cannot engage in dialogue. Cannot retell a story and give picture description. Can repeat words and short sentences, sometimes echolalic but cannot alter order. Can initiate novel answer if given visual cue. Writing may be grammatically accurate but meaningless. Reduced awareness of errors.

produce word-substitution errors and gross lesions to the left temporal lobe destroy the lexicon.

Recent cerebral blood flow and positron emission tomography studies have reinforced a classic localisation of areas of language and brain function. Such areas work in functional concert. The right hemisphere, far from being silent, metabolises more diffusely than the left in the comprehension and verbalisation of language. Wernicke's area monitors verbalised language continually, although automatic speech is less dramatically monitored. The region of the supplementary motor area is identified as a programmer of language in both thought and expression. The overlapping areas of the parietal, temporal and occipital areas are also thought to be involved in cross-modal processing. Reading and writing, or the transcoding of phonemes to graphemes, metabolises complex pathways and the association areas of the posterior cortex. Since the posterior brain is more likely to be affected by ageing the greatest errors in language would appear to be disruptions of naming, complex auditory processing and phonemic decoding. Indeed, many of the 'dysarthric' errors noted in the speech of the elderly may result from faulty central processing.

The most subtle language changes are comprehension deficits. Impaired comprehension in the aged may relate to deafness or to an auditory processing component as discrimination or perception of temporal and competing stimuli. Comprehension may also be a result of a loss of auditory memory, or the ability to hold information while it is being processed. The medial and inferior temporal lobes are responsible for verbal memory and undergo neurological change in normal ageing. This produces a diminished immediate memory which is demonstrated by the decline of digit recall scores quite dramatically after the eighth decade. In anteriograde amnesia the elderly may hold the final piece of information, and in retrograde amnesia they will only recall initial information. This inability to hold information may lead to a failure of cohesion in expressive language, where references to component parts of sentences lose the ties that make utterances unified.

Failure of syntactic analysis of the elderly has been reported in language assessments as Part F of the Token Test, which demands comprehension of complex instructions where sentence length is held constant and redundancy eliminated, and by psycholinguistic studies that have investigated compensatory strategies the elderly employ in the face of a failure of syntactic analysis. By the seventh decade the elderly have greater difficulty understanding inference, anomaly and ambiguity. They are less able to recall propositional information and rely on semantic information to understand rather than process complex linguistic forms. This deterioration in established comprehension has brought under review the concept of 'crystalline' versus 'fluid' abilities or the dichotomy of language learnt against language learning. Tasks that demand definition and comprehension are usually considered crystalline and represent stable information, and tasks that demand flexibility are fluid and reflect the functioning neurological system. In age these two concepts are dissociated. This can be demonstrated by comparing the discrepancy that increases in the scores of an index of crystalline ability, the WAIS vocabulary, and fluid ability, the Matrices of Raven, that measure verbal reasoning.

Semantic knowledge as word meaning tested by definition is relatively stable in ageing, hence the greater resilience of convergent verbal tasks over divergent verbal tasks as the generation of word strings. This failure to generate tasks of word fluency suggests that active vocabulary diminishes while passive or recognition vocabulary remains. This dichotomy between word knowledge and word usage can also be explained in terms of crystalline and fluid intelligence.

Investigations by linguistic analysis may be compared with neurolinguistic studies. Changes in language usage may be subtle, since the elderly change strategies to compensate and enhance functional communication skills. These attempts may produce adverse effects. 'Chronic senile loquacity', marked by increased word counts, may be an attempt to mask impairment much like the confabulation of Korsakoff psychosis or jargon in Wernicke's aphasia. Even those with dementia, who have difficulty generating novel word lists, will produce those words at normal frequency over time in their discourse.

The aged use more words, more fillers and more dysfluencies. They also use fewer total sentences and generate fewer themes. There are pausological effects, fewer embedded sentences, more sentences left unfinished, a greater range of indefinite words, more pronouns than proper nouns and more nouns turned into verb forms similar to the verbal paraphasia seen in Wernicke's aphasia. These difficulties that arise in the spontaneous use of language may relate to language planning and reduced semantics and syntactic abilities. By comparison, when writing the elderly produce well-structured full sentences with complex syntax.

Several tests of neurolinguistic ability have demonstrated that 15 per cent of the normal population will produce linguistic errors characteristic of dysphasia or dementia. One Glasgow study (Walker, 1982) demonstrated that a healthy normal aged population divided into five-year bands from the sixth to the eighth decades will produce an increase of percentage errors in writing, visuomotor, auditory, language and reading skills. A similar Edinburgh study (Thompson, 1986) correlated a wide range of neurolinguistic and non-verbal tasks of intelligence to normal ageing, and found that the healthy elderly were significantly impaired in both the ability to retrieve names, generate abstract word lists, comprehend instructions and repeat sentence and number streams of increasing length. There is also a rise in the motor programming aspect of speech as an oral apraxia. More significantly impaired is their ability to spell, which is probably related to transcoding deficits in the posterior cortex. Most significantly related to ageing are the abilities that demand visuospatial processes that, as complexity increases, are increasingly verbally mediated. Tasks such as Block Design and Calculation fall into this category.

THE LANGUAGE OF DEMENTIA

The problem of mild dementia in neurolinguistic analysis is to define which errors are pathological and which are not. It is estimated that 80 per cent of the healthy population will make cognitive errors assigned to 'benign senescent forgetfulness' and 15 per cent will go on to make pathological errors. This grey area of normal to abnormal ageing has provoked the argument that dementia may be an acceleration of the ageing process.

Miller (1981) has noted that research in dementia has focused on memory disturbance, and that there has been little on language disturbance and less on perception, information processing, visuospatial ability and thinking. There have been several descriptions of the general features of language in dementia. They describe a lack of verbal spontaneity and speech initiative with a slowness or a refusal to respond. Generally the language of the demented is considered circuitous, vague and empty but fluent. Echolalia is more common than mutism, and both are a late feature of the disorder.

It is generally considered that the naming errors made by those with a dementia are lost hierarchically and similar to the paraphasias found in Wernicke-type aphasia. Naming errors are well documented and relate either to a loss of vocabulary or failure to access it. There has also been an argument that naming errors are a result of an agnosia or a failure to visually perceive the object to be named. All such errors are common to lesions of the tertiary cortex where the temporal parietal and occipital areas overlap.

The result of anomia is that language becomes 'empty'. Nouns are selectively lost rather than adjectives, pronouns, prepositions and conjunctions. Abstract nouns are more vulner-

131

able than concrete ones and the loss of nouns relates to their frequency in the lexicon. People with dementia are more likely to use vague generalisations like 'thing', rather than search for appropriate labels. They are more likely to attempt to stabilise their fading lexicon by adding personal possessive labels such as 'my tie' or 'your pen', or make nouns more concrete by providing verbal labels such as 'drawing pencil' or 'drinking cup'. This suggests the use of verbal paraphasias to aid the search for nouns. It is this loosening of semantic ties and concept formation that produces a loss of the associated links of words, and the things they represent, which produces speech without content.

Word fluency and ideational fluency as tested by the ability to generate word strings starting with a given letter, or word strings of object classifications, decrease in dementia, although in measures of oral fluency of normal spontaneous speech, words that occur infrequently in word strings are normally distributed in discourse.

Naming tasks have been used to diagnose dementing processes. Several authors have noticed increased latency of naming, that the degree of naming parallels the degree of dementia and that naming skills may have the ability to differentiate alcoholic dementia from Alzheimer and vascular dementia. On group data language tasks have not been able to differentiate Alzheimer-type dementia from multi-infarct dementia, although differences may occur in individual cases.

The reason for the breakdown of semantic fields remains unclear. It may represent a failure of a 'law of strength', the pathological brain being unable to select from competing stimuli so that weak stimuli arouse strong associations and this lack of selectivity produced paraphasia. Perhaps the redundancy of language in dementia may be a result of the individual's need to qualify lexemes in unsteady and diminishing fields, so the ability to make broad classifications is retained, but the ability to make more precise selection within semantic fields is lost. A third possibility is the dual representation of names. Visual engrams may be matched to verbal analogues of concrete but not abstract nouns. A misaligning of an auditory analogue to a visual engram has been interpreted as producing the agnosic component in anomia. The suggestion has been raised that whereas aphasia is a difficulty of access and retrieval of nouns, dementia is a difficulty of recognition. However, dementing people can often gesture the use of objects they cannot name and be phonetically cued. This suggests that they do have an internal representation of objects they cannot label, and that those labels are not so much lost but less accessible.

Phonemic paraphasias are sound substitution errors, and are rarer than semantic paraphasia or word substitution errors. Semantic paraphasia includes circumlocution, generic terms and terms of vague reference. The semantic paraphasias found with dementing individuals are unlike those of aphasics and tend to involve greater use of circumlocution (see Table 5.2).

Logoclonia, echolalia and perseveration, but seldom mutism, have been described in dementia. Intrusion errors enter the discourse of 89 per cent of patients with Alzheimer's disease. These intrusion errors, or learned words, are unrelated to specific tasks but perseverate into discourse as a distinguishing feature of Alzheimer's disease. The number of intrusions is shown to be sensitive to cholinergic therapy. However, intrusions occur in multiple-infarct dementia and aphasia where perseveration is far more common.

Syntactic errors may be agrammatic, where utterances are short with the omission of function words, or paragrammatic, as fluent and copious speech with function words and affixes often misused. Discohesive speech is a failure of sentences, clauses and phrases to relate to each other by lexical reference. Loss of cohesion has been described in the language of schizophrenia and normal ageing but not in the language of dementia. This area needs to be systematically investigated, for while it appears generally true that syntax is more resistant to semantics, the loss of immediate memory in dementia appears to produce a failure of sequenced discourse.

Selective impairment of semantic memory would suggest that grammar and the lexicon are independent. There may be a filter for grammatical structures that is independent of cognition, or grammar may be more tightly wired than semantics. Repetition studies have shown that grammar is preserved at the expense of syntax and that those with a dementia are able to correct errors of morphology. They may not be asyntactic listeners like Broca's aphasics, but may be like the normal elderly who are forced to rely on context to comprehend. There is evidence from the writing of Alzheimer-type patients that they misperceive phonological markers and therefore may act on only the gist of what they hear (Thompson, 1986).

Table 5.2: Naming errors in mild, moderate and severe Alzheimer-type dementia

Target	Nominal paraphasia	Verbal paraphasia	Circumlocution
Moderate dementia: naming errors			
Razor	razor blade	shaver	to cut hair
			for doing your face
			for shaving
Tweezers	pincers	pluckers	cut eyebrows
	nippers	clippers	to clear splinters
	pliers		
Bell	gong		to call with it
			ring
			put it to work
Gun			shoot
			kids play with it
Sponge			for washing yourself
			thing for washing
Torch	lamp	lighter	flash thing
	lantern		
Moderate dementia: naming errors			
Pen	propelling pencil		for writing
			an old type of nib
Matches	cigarettes		smoke them
Cup	jug		tea or coffee
Whistle	rattle		
Paintbrush			for teeth
Severe dementia: naming errors			
Torch	battery		flashing
Razor		shaver	the man shave
			for your face
Pipe			put things in it
			to stuff it in and puff
Pen	pencil		
	pointed cane		
Sponge			soft
Watch	clock		
Scissors			cutting
			you have long nails
Cup			eating
			drinking
			eat from it
Whistle	bell		put in mouth
Bell	whistle		to make a noise
Brush			for painting
Glasses			speak
			to look at
			for eyes
Fork			cooking

Grammatical errors exist in dementia, a proportion of sentences and phrases are incomplete, there is a loss of plural markers and grammatical non-agreement that may be interpreted as a loss of short-term memory with resultant loss of cohesion.

The loss of the use of language, or its pragmatics, has also been noted in dementia. Communication is often stimulus-bound, there is a reliance on context and reduced ability to generate novel utterances. With the loss of speech initiative and the restriction of language to statements and requests there is a loss of questioning. This pragmatic divorce is between language and the purpose it represents. A hallmark of the difference of the language of aphasia and dementia may be that those with aphasia attempt to communicate a message whereas dementing individuals may no longer know what the message is.

The penultimate stage of language deterioration in the demented, preceding mutism, appears to be repetition, substitution and perseveration of verbal stereotypes. Speech is reduced to syllabic palilalia that has been described following intellectual deterioration with bilateral lesions. It represents an endless repetition of syllable, word and phrases both verbally and graphically. It has been indexed to linguistic decline just as linguistic decline in dementia has been indexed to death.

Some authorities have described the language of dementia in terms of aphasia, and many authors have noted linguistic errors in normal ageing that are similar to the errors produced by focal and diffuse lesions. In 1892 Pick described his patient as presenting transcortical sensory aphasia, while Alzheimer described aphasia and paraphasia in his patient of 1907. The empty speech of Alzheimer's disease is not characteristic of the neologism that accompanies Wernicke's aphasia, but it may be similar to the semantic aphasias that reflect posterior parietal involvement in that it is usually fluent and with a reduction of content words. There is little evidence of comprehension deficits in early dementia related to a failure to decode speech sounds, and little evidence of expressive phonemic disturbance. Oddly enough a phonemic disturbance may be reflected in the writing of Alzheimer-type patients who produce graphemic substitution errors not dissimilar to those found in the speech of mild Wernicke's aphasics (see Figure 5.1).

Good arguments exist for the independence of aphasia and dementing language. Aphasia is of sudden onset, and follows circumscribed lesions to the left hemisphere. Aphasics generally improve their linguistic performance, or their communicative performance, with management. Factorial studies have shown that the psychological clustering of abilities in neurolinguistic data from dementing and aphasic clients is different (Hodkinson, Stevens and Kenny, 1984; Thompson, 1986). Language is lost late in the progression of Alzheimer-type dementia and only a few studies have reported it as a presenting feature. Finally language loss in dementia is a result of diffuse lesions and is slow and insidious in its history (see Figure 5.1).

There are weaknesses in most studies of the language of dementia. There are few longitudinal studies and many reports are clinical impressions without scientific methodology. There is an assumption that language following focal lesions can be validly compared to language following generalised lesions. Many studies define language in terms of verbal intelligence and use multifactorial tests in their investigation. Studies have been conducted with different aims that bias methodology and results; some have attempted to compare language breakdown in adults with language acquisition in children and some have attempted to produce a grammar of the demented. It is important that future studies have experimental groups that are tightly defined, that language as a communicative performance is investigated longitudinally and that tests are developed that are specific to the effects of the diseases being examined.

LANGUAGE AND COGNITION

The relationship of language to cognition and thought remains unclear. Cognition involves the ability to perceive, analyse, select, store, synthesise and retrieve information. Language is a symbolic system that allows and facilitates this achievement. Childhood autism has been described as a failure in childhood to develop a language system as a tool to their cognition. Studies of both adult and child cognitive processes have shown the use of subvocalisation in cognitive processing to be valuable in the role of the solution of complex problems.

'Intelligence' is the measurement of selective cognitive abilities, and may be impaired in aphasia. It is certainly reduced in dementia and selectively reduced in normal ageing. The decline of the mean scores of both verbal and non-verbal sections of the WAIS and the more rapid and early decline of visuospatial abilities over verbal intelligence is an index of declining intelligence in normal ageing.

A failure of specific cognitive ability in ageing has been related to increasing neuronal impairment. Thirty to forty per cent of the healthy elderly demonstrate slowing of the EEG, while reduced metabolism measured by blood flow and metabolic studies is confirmed over the frontotemporal areas. Neuropathological studies in normal ageing show selective atrophy in the superior temporal gyrus. The loquaciousness and garrulousness of ageing may be associated with cortical and subcortical changes.

Cortical functioning in abstract cognitive tasks has been best described by *in vivo* studies using cerebral blood flow and positron emission tomography. Levels of thinking as reflected by increased flow depend on the nature of the task. Cognitive processing demands increased cerebral flow with specific metabolism of the posterior cortex. In particular, tasks that require abstract problem-solving, rearrangement of data or concentration — such as digit repetition in reverse and the Progressive Matrices of Raven — cause higher global flow.

Studies in the normal activation of speech, reading and problem-solving have indicated that in listening there is increased bilateral flow over the auditory cortex and Wernicke's area which mediates the understanding of speech. In speech there is increased flow over the articulatory areas of the motor and sensory cortex as well as the temporoparietal cortex, the supplementary motor area and the inferior areas of the frontal lobes.

Automatic speech makes fewer demands on language by being non-propositional. Tests that ask for mental effort increase flow over the temporo-occipital regions and temporal regions, which are known to be involved in highly integrated sensory activities as well as in hearing and auditory memory. The frontal motor speech areas are utilised in conscious intellectual processes and logical operations. The Progressive Matrices of Raven are reasoning tests that involve visual perception and complex analysis of given problems by subvocal analogy. When the solution is found the result is verbalised. Thus in addition to problem-solving the test involves verbal functions including covert 'inner' speech.

137

The upper convexity of the frontal lobe and supplementary motor areas appears to have a specific role in the planning and regulation of linguistic tasks. This suggests the role of the supplementary motor area is a programmer of dynamic movements. Fluency is disturbed in frontal lobe disease, and in particular the left supplementary motor area appears to have a role in verbal rather than ideational fluency.

Psychological tests that demand abstract thinking involve the association cortex. In Alzheimer dementia these areas are functionally low at rest; in fact there is deactivation during psychological testing and reading. This failure of activity has been called 'intellectual steal' and may relate to dementing individuals attempting to use different strategies, for example not seeing an abstract reasoning test as a problem but simply perceiving it, and thereby inducing greater activity of the primary sensory regions. Alzheimer patients with expressive and receptive language disturbances have reduced flow in temporal and occipital areas but not precentral areas. People with Pick's disease who are unable to regulate their linguistic behaviour show temporofrontal lobe deficiencies, again with central areas spared.

Neuropsychological tests that tap intellectual abilities, such as Block Design, are multifactorial. They demand sustained attention, visuospatial thought, motor assembly and the role of language in analysing a problem, planning its solution and monitoring the outcome. There is little wonder that Block Design is sensitive to early dementia. Which abilities within the conglomerate of skills needed to complete such a task are most sensitive is speculative. Some psychologists have argued that subtests of the WAIS such as Verbal Similarities are more sensitive, and that it is linguistic as much as visuospatial deficits that are impaired in all stages of dementia. Certainly tests that demand subvocalisation and abstract processing demonstrate continually reducing scores in both normal and abnormal ageing. Tests that are not standardised but demand abstract sorting such as the Weigl Colour Form Sorting Test, produce progressive deterioration of scores in the healthy elderly (Walker, 1982).

Coupled with a loss of cognitive ability and verbal language is the increasing loss of paralinguistic communication. The role of interpersonal space (proxemics), gesture (kinesics), gaze and pause phenomena all provide for the social setting of human interaction, turn-taking, dynamism and regulation of inter-loquacionary acts. While this paralinguistic behaviour has created a great deal of attention in terms of social biology there are few reported studies of psychosocial linguistics. There has been considerable interest in the management of the dementing in communicative settings, or the adapting of the environment to patients' deficits in reality orientation programmes, institutional normalisation and therapeutic or prosthetic environments. Human communication studies of the effects of decreased affect and the loss of gaze phenomena that accompanies the flat basal stare of the demented, increasing limb apraxia that disturbs kinesis, and the failure of insight that regulates socially appropriate space would be a rewarding study for students of social and institutional behaviour.

HEARING IMPAIRMENT

The greatest deficit of communication in normal ageing is hearing loss or presbycusis. It may begin from the third to the fifth decade and be a cumulative effect of inner ear changes, noise pollution and toxicity. High-frequency signals are particularly impaired, and this loss of sensitivity may occur in conjunction with the loss of cognitive processes such as concentration, and a decline of central linguistic performance. High-frequency bands are vital to speech perception because these frequencies carry consonants and formant transitions of vowels. Consonants have smaller temporal duration than vowels, and the elderly are less able to process the temporal aspect of speech. The position is exacerbated because the elderly are less able to attend to competing stimuli that, as background noise, masks speech. This failure of speech perception begins in the fifth decade and accelerates to the seventh. Loss of hearing acuity is coupled with diminished speech discrimination. Social inadequacy in adults may occur with mild hearing loss from 40 to 50 dB, and measurable psychological problems are often apparent in moderate loss from 55 to 70 dB. Carers report that hearing loss produces social and emotional problems of inadequacy, isolation and paranoia, particularly in institutional settings where seating and management procedures make patients passive responders to their environment.

The combination of increasingly diminished hearing loss

affecting comprehension of verbo-acoustic signals and the decreasing ability of the posterior cortex to analyse language at sound and syntactic level, together with a deterioration of the temporoparietal cortex and the frontolimbic area, produces diminished comprehension of the linguistic environment with a rise of loquacity and communicative inappropriateness. The combined effect for the elderly is increasing isolation, rejection, shame and bewilderment. It is a pity therefore, that far more is known about the breakdown of communication in the elderly than how such processes may be managed.

THE MANAGEMENT OF COMMUNICATION DISORDERS IN ELDERLY PEOPLE

The assessment of cognitive disorders and communication disorders in the elderly is the responsibility of psychologists, neuropsychologists, audiologists and speech pathologists. The management of such disorders is traditionally the responsibility of the speech pathologist. Their role is the diagnosis and description of deficits of voice, speech and language. They instigate therapeutic regimes, counsel clients and their families, provide in-service education, liaise with the community and other professionals and act as a resource for staff and administration. Their skills are interrelated with audiologists and hearing therapists in aural rehabilitation, physiotherapists and medical staff in the management of swallowing disorders and with occupational therapists in reading and writing deficits.

Aural rehabilitation

Seven per cent of the general population, and over 40 per cent of the population over 75 years old are hearing-impaired. The deficits are related to auditory processing, communication and the psychosocial difficulties of depression and withdrawal that may be consequent upon them.

Peripheral hearing loss may be caused by local inflammation, impacted cerumen or perforation of the eardrum. Middle ear disorders may result from otosclerosis or fixation of the stapes to the cochlea window. It may also result from decreased articulation of the ossicles or otitis media following Eustachian tube malfunction. Presbycusis generally results from cochlea or retrocochlea disease. In the cochlea, hair cells determine the frequency of acoustic signals. The information is carried by the auditory nerve to the auditory cortex. Presbycusis may be a combined result of age, noise and the effects of ototoxic drugs. Hearing loss in the elderly is often specifically related to high-frequency sounds. This accounts for the difficulty they have hearing telephones and doorbells. In speech many consonants are also identified by higher frequency, so information in speech signals is not perceived.

The assessment of hearing loss involves pure tone audiometry and measures speech reception and discrimination. Aural rehabilitation includes both supplying and orientation of hearing aids, but provision depends upon the type of hearing loss, the personality of the wearer, ability to care for moulds and dexterity in tuning the apparatus. Hearing aids are not as cosmetically acceptable as glasses and, in spite of improved orientation, many still find their way into drawers and lockers. Aural rehabilitation also includes auditory training, lip-reading skills and the use of paralinguistic language to convey information. Comprehension is heightened in the hearing-impaired, such as the speaker's need to face the listener, neither shouting nor speaking in the ear of the client, maintaining normal speech rates, not over-articulating nor concealing the mouth in speech, as well as organising seating, lighting and social settings to provide optimum visual information. Intervention that is early may overcome the negative effects of age, adaptability and habit.

Voice and speech rehabilitation

Voice and speech disorders are a result of reduced breathing patterns, phonation, articulation, resonance and prosody disorders. Ventilatory capacity of the lungs is reduced by smoking and posture. Habitual clavicular breathing patterns with a loss of central diaphragmatic breathing decrease the amount of air available for sustained speech. Capacity is reduced in ageing females by postural effects of osteoporosis.

Disorders of voice in ageing are caused and sustained by habitual hyperfunction and poor vocal hygiene. Smoking and dusty atmospheres, and musculoskeletal tension, are also common causes of dysphonia. Sudden changes in swallowing or

141

vocal quality may reflect organic lesions and should be reported to otolaryngologists.

Age effects on speech patterns result from fatigue and diminished strength and elasticity. Articulation is effected by loss of dentition, ill-fitting dentures, decreased tissue bulk and changes in the alignment of the jaw. These changes affect the shape and speed of tongue movement; they also affect the ability of the articulatory apparatus to form consonants. Nevertheless speech patterns in the elderly generally remain adequate. Vowels carry the acoustic information rather than consonants. Syntax is rule-governed and therefore predictable. Speech is both repetitious and redundant, and can be supplemented by a wide range of paralinguistic information including writing, spelling, gesture, gaze, facial affect, pause, vocalisation, topic and context. Obvious ageing speech deficits are low volume and a loss of prosodic contours. These patterns are particularly noted as secondary to the dementing process in vascular dementia and in Parkinsonism.

The role of the speech pathologist in speech disorders is to define systemic dysfunction in paralysis, weakness, abnormality of tone, and loss of speed, dynamism or co-ordination. Specific disorders demand specific therapies, including relaxation, postural manipulation, phrasing, oral exercises, the use of prosodic features to compensate loss of articulatory skills and stimulation by proprioceptive techniques.

Language rehabilitation

Disturbances of language or aphasia need to be identified from dysarthria, apraxia of speech (which is a motor programming disorder) and the language of affective, confusional and cognitive states. Language may be a part of a wider dementing syndrome, or it may exist as an aphasia, following focal infarction in stroke, neoplastic disease or vascular dementia. Speech pathologists therefore need to examine language function in terms of cognitive disruption, its effect on a client's activities of daily living, and whether language deficits will improve.

Assessments must be valid, reliable and discriminating, describing specific deficits and differentiating disease processes. Deficits may include agnosia, the failure of perception of auditory and visual stimuli, or apraxia. Apraxias are disturbances of volitional programming. They can impair articulatory movement, gesture and operations in three-dimensional space.

Comprehension deficits result from a loss of hearing acuity, reduced auditory memory, faulty speech perception, impaired phonemic decoding, or an inability to analyse words or grammar. Language errors include phonemic and semantic paraphasias where sounds or words are substituted within a similar category. Studies in semantic processing investigate whether words are actually lost or whether the problem is one of retrieval. Syntactic errors may be agrammatic in telegraphic speech or paragrammatic with errors of morphological markers or suffixes. In wider discourse there may be a loss of cohesion and reference, which is a diminution of the relationship of words and clauses within a sentence.

Symbolic language disorders relate to reading, writing and calculation. The most subtle reading dissociation is between oral reading and comprehension. Writing disorders, or dysgraphias, reflect deficits of verbal language as dyssyntactic or orthographic dysgraphia, or they may reflect a visuospatial disorder such as calligraphic dysgraphia. Calculation reflects visuospatial deficits and a reduced ability to use language in abstract problem-solving. This role of language may be observed in tests of non-verbal intelligence which demand visuospatial processing as well as the ability to reason by subvocal analogy or the ability to monitor motor behaviour with language.

The management of language disorders is only as precise as assessment, but is based on both facilitation and enhancement of communicative proficiency. Remediation of comprehension disorders involves tasks of phonemic discrimination or the ability to differentiate between single words whose meaning is altered by a single sound or feature such as voicing, manner and articulatory placement. Further procedures demand identifying meaning by word order and semantic markers. Management of expressive language disorders is tailored to break down at different levels of processing. Remediation of naming skills, for example, would involve the deficit as one of semantic loss, access or retrieval, and therefore demand definition or retraining of word meaning, cueing by sound and word association or the use of forced alternatives.

Agrammaticism is managed by identifying sentence tasks in terms of grammatical categories and combining them sequentially. Paragrammatic errors and loss of function words are restored by tasks that demand sentence construction, sentence completion and techniques using tag questions to generate responses without repetition or echoing. Recent developments in aphasia therapy have been outlined by Code and Muller (1983), while the enhancement of functional communication in aphasics has been described by Chapey (1981) and Davis (1980). The development of PACE (the promotion of aphasic communicative effectiveness) has modified therapeutic strategies. There is an increase in turn-taking, the need for both client and therapist to be less familiar with messages to encourage the use of as many modalities and channels of communication as possible. This emphasis on modality and paralinguistics in communication has followed assessments of functional communication published by Holland (1982) and Skinner, Wirz, Thompson and Davidson (1984).

Recent methods of management of aphasia have employed linguistic models of information processing at acoustic/ phonemic, semantic/pragmatic and syntactic/thematic representations. Emphasis is placed on the intention and message as pragmatics and this dichotomy between an intended message, and an apparent loss of communicative intent appears to be a difference in aphasia and the language of the demented. Emphasis is also placed on how linguistic units are analysed, stored and retrieved. Models of information processing are derived from logogen systems and have been elaborated after Morton (1985).

More specific techniques of communication restoration include melodic intonation therapy for articulatory dyspraxia, which uses the musicality of the brain to assist verbalisation by manipulating pitch, melody and voice quality to convey meaning. Visual action therapy has been used for global aphasia where symbolic gestures communicate reference and elements of grammar. More recently aphasia treatment and microcomputers have received attention in terms of software and the role of computers in clinical research and therapy developments (Katz, 1986). Microcomputers have allowed the establishing of language restoration programmes that are self-directing.

The efficacy of aphasia therapy has prompted controversial studies in recent years. The overall conclusions are that aphasics improve in the initial twelve months post-onset. Treated aphasics do better than those that are not treated. Trained volunteers are effective but need to be guided by speech pathologists.

144

Treatment delay does not hinder the results of language therapy, but remediation ought to begin in the first few months after onset for the most significant improvements to occur. Prognostic indicators appear to be aetiology, severity, site and size of lesion, management, motivation and improvements in other areas such as mobility. Neither age nor intelligence appears to be a factor in language rehabilitation.

There are then several principles relating to the management of language impairment in the elderly. These principles differ in the management of aphasia and non-aphasia-producing lesions. There are, however, some similarities. Language works by inter-action, and the problem of a breakdown of communication lies with the listener as well as the speaker. Language loss may be a problem of access, and therefore communication needs to be facilitated as well as taught. Language assessment and manage-ment ought to be non-threatening and functional. Language therapy may be both investigative and rehabilitative. Language needs to be kept simple, and information presented in discrete units while facilitation strategies need to be enhanced paralin-guistically to convey as much information as possible across all modalities.

Cognitive rehabilitation

Cognition is the perception, transformation, storage and retrie-val of information. Language is a vehicle for these processes and represents the achievement of cognition. Immediate or auditory memory is involved in comprehension loss both in acoustic amnesic aphasia and the language pathology of Alzheimer-type dementia. In both these conditions the basal temporal lobes are affected, and memory traces are not strong enough to hold information while it is being processed. Information is lost and in verbal expression language may lose cohesion. Recent memory is impaired in dementia. Generally long-term memory is preserved in both disorders. The language-impaired are usually able to remember their birth date and birth place because that is stable information that never changes. Ribot's Law states that the most durable memories are the longest, and this principle has been the basis of reminiscence therapy and the skilful use of nostalgia to encourage communication in geriatric groups. The practical reason for this is that the elderly are a product of memories which need enhancing. The elderly demented are increasingly impaired in their learning, and demonstrate a dissociation between word and word meaning, but the use of signposting, trails and reality orientation has demonstrated that aspects of behaviour and language can be successfully manipulated.

Disturbances of language and cognition can also accompany affective disorders such as pseudodementia. Pseudodementia can be managed by a course of antidepressants, but skilled neurolinguistic periodic testing can plot the course of improvement with drug therapy (see Figure 5.2). Depressed patients are able to life their scores with the therapist's encouragement, unlike organic dementias where patients are unable to improve their responses. Neurolinguistic assessment in affective and organic dementia may have a role. The assessments are non-threatening and demonstrate patterns of behaviour that differ in the inexorable decline of language in Alzheimer's disease or focal neurological pathology of vascular diagnosis of organic and non-organic dementia which are commonly confused.

The role of speech pathology

Speech pathologists have been more concerned with disorders of voice, fluency and language development than in the breakdown of language and communication in ageing and dementia. Demographic changes in western industrialised countries will demand more research on ageing communication impairments. Little is published on the management of communication disorders in the dementing and the healthy ageing population, and therapists' management programmes are often very skilful and practical but not published. The lack of knowledge on ageing and care is reflected in the few chairs of geriatric medicine, the fewer chairs in psychogeriatric medicine and the lack of chairs in gerontology, the sociological and psychological problems of the aged. The elderly are increasingly institutionalised but the long-term effects of hospitalisation are not known. It is disturbing that language impairment is positively related to long-term care, and the degree of language pathology is related to mortality.

Therapists need to develop their tests, and select materials and patients and methods for optimum management in order to investigate the most effective communicative strategies of remediation. At the same time wider issues of management of communication disorders such as appropriateness of lifestyle and the relationship of other handicaps such as mobility, dementia and sensory deficits, have to be considered. In this regard therapists need to create a therapeutic environment.

Environmental changes themselves produce confusion in the elderly, such as in housing relocation with its loss of social contacts and interaction. Too often the elderly present to their GPs following such events and are sedated. This in turn produces greater disorientation, such that the elderly increasingly present at hospital casualty departments to be labelled acute brain syndrome. Speech therapists need to be able to distinguish between the transient language of confusion and language pathology consequent upon organic changes. There is a real need for a quick screening procedure to differentiate acute and chronic brain syndromes.

Speech pathologists need to be involved in institutional care and counsel on appropriate hospitalisation, day care, nursing home accommodation and community services. They need to advise on whether the best communicative settings are community-based, and in institutionalised settings create a stimulating communicative environment that provides optimum normalisation and independence and are relevant, sensitive, interactive, accepting and appropriate. They need to investigate which therapeutic strategies are best related to the adaptability of the ageing brain, whether group or individual management is preferable, and how best to enhance language as an instrument in the everyday needs of their clients.

Finally, speech pathologists need to establish a role in counselling the family and professional carers on which aspects of communication are impaired, and whether insight and intelligence are retained.

The tragedy of failure of precise diagnosis of speech and language disorders in both normal and abnormal ageing is reflected in aphasic patients committed to long-term wards with the demented. Their cognitive ability is more intact, and their plight can be compared to that of Zola's Madam Raquin:

Walled in intelligence, still alive yet imprisoned in dead flesh ... she could see, hear, and doubtless she could reason quite clearly. Yet she had no movement or speech to express her

Figure 5.1: Test profile of a client with Alzheimer's disease

NAME
SEX   Female
D of B   Age 57 years
DIAGNOSIS   Alzheimer Type Dementia

DATE 6.2.82
– – – – 2.9.83
——— 13.1.84

PERCENTILES

TEST	MAX. SCORE	<5	10	20	30	40	50	60	70	80	90	95<
RATING SCALE	40	9	13	17	20	22	24 25	26	27	30	32	35 8
IDENTIFICATION/NAME	8		7									8
IDENTIFICATION/FUNCTION	8	6	7									8
TOKEN TEST Part A–E	67		47	52	57	60	62		63		65 66	67
TOKEN TEST Part F	96		56	66	69	76	81 85	86	87	89	91	95
TOKEN TEST Total	163	92	114	126 129	133	139	147	148	152		159	162
SENTENCE REPETITION	22	9	8	10	11		12	13			14	
REPEATING DIGITS	14		3	4	5		6		7		8	
REPEATING DIGITS REVERSE	14		1	2	3		4		5			
AUTOMATIC SPEECH	4		2		3							4
CONFRONTATION NAMING	16		12		14		14 15					16
DESCRIPTION OF FUNCTION	16		15									16
TACTILE NAMING (Right)	8		5	6			7					8
TACTILE NAMING (Left)	8		5	6		7						8

148

Profile chart (percentile scale along horizontal axis): **<5   10   20   30   40   50   60   70   80   90   95<**

Test	Max	Plotted scores
FLUENCY	60	0, 4, 6, 7, 8, 9, 10, 11, 12, 13, 17, 23
SENTENCE CONSTRUCTION	25	0, 3, 6, 9, 12, 4, 17, 19, 22, 23, 25
READING WORDS	8	7, 8
WORD RECOGNITION	8	7, 8
READING SENTENCES	7	3, 7
SENTENCE COMPREHENSION	32	8, 20, 21, 24, 25, 27, 28, 29, 31, 32
AUTOMATIC WRITING	5	2, 4, 5
SPELLING	24	9, 13, 16, 21, 22, 24
DICTATION	13	8, 10, 11, 12, 13
COPYING	11	6, 7, 8, 9, 10, 11
CALCULATION	10	4, 6, 7, 8, 10
ORAL	20	16, 19, 20
IDEOMOTOR	20	14, 16, 17, 18, 19, 20
CONSTRUCTIONAL	20	8, 10, 11, 16, 17, 19, 20
BLOCK DESIGN	48	0, 4, 6, 8, 11, 16, 17, 20
RAVEN'S MATRICES	36	10, 14, 16, 17, 18, 20, 23, 25

Comment: The assessments show increasing disintegration of cognitive ability. There is an early loss of memory contaminating auditory comprehension. Semantic skills were retained, but intrusion-errors noted as dementia fell from mild to moderate. Reading was dissociated from understanding, and writing ability deteriorated, as did the ability of complex calculation. Constructional abilities were progressively lost and measures of intelligence progressively diminished.

149

Figure 5.2: Test profile of a client with pseudo-dementia

NAME

SEX Male

D of B Age 68 years

DIAGNOSIS Pseudo-dementia

DATE 29.4.84

- - - - - 1.2.85

TEST	MAX. SCORE	5	10	20	30	40	50	60	70	80	90	95
						PERCENTILES						
RATING SCALE	40	(36)	(38)									40
IDENTIFICATION/NAME	8		7									(8)
IDENTIFICATION/FUNCTION	8		7									(8)
TOKEN TEST Part A–E	67	64	65		(66)							(67)
TOKEN TEST Part F	96		90	(92)			95					(96)
TOKEN TEST Total	163		154	(159)	160		(162)					163
SENTENCE REPETITION	22		12			14	15	16	17	(18)	(19)	20
REPEATING DIGITS	14		5		6		7	(8)	9	(10)	11	12
REPEATING DIGITS REVERSE	14	3	4	5	(6)		(7)	8	9	10		12
AUTOMATIC SPEECH	4											(4)
CONFRONTATION NAMING	16	14				15						(16)
DESCRIPTION OF FUNCTION	16		10									(16)
TACTILE NAMING (Right)	8				7							(8)
TACTILE NAMING (Left)	8				7							(8)
GESTURE	16	16										(16)
FLUENCY	60	(8) (12)	20	27	31	33	35	36	40	44	50	60

Test											Score
READING WORDS	8										(8)
WORD RECOGNITION	8										(8)
READING SENTENCES	7										7
SENTENCE COMPREHENSION	32										32 · (31)
AUTOMATIC WRITING	5										(5)
SPELLING	24	(21)		(23)							24
DICTATION	13	11	12								(13)
COPYING	11	9	10								(11)
CALCULATION	10	8	9								(10)
ORAL	20										(20)
IDEOMOTOR	20										(20)
CONSTRUCTIONAL	20	18	19								(20)
BLOCK DESIGN	48	15	(20)	(24)	25	27	28	30	35	40	42
RAVEN'S MATRICES	36	19	20	23	(25)	27	28	(29)	31	33	34 35	36
		5	10	20	30	40	50	60	70	80	90 95

Comment: Depression affecting cognitive performance and masquerading as dementia is well recognised. The condition is often labelled 'pseudodementia'. A differential diagnosis is critical, the conditions of organic and nonorganic dementias have different treatments and different outcomes. At least 15 per cent of the elderly depressed will present cognitive deficits that can include language and memory disturbance. Affective disorders are also described in dementing populations. Aphasias, apraxias and agnosias are rare in depression. Depressed patients do not perseverate and are subject to lability. Many cognitive deficits resolve with antidepressants. In this profile, unlike those of degenerative dementias, scores have generally remained stable.

thoughts to the outside world. Maybe her thoughts choked her ... Her mind was like one of those people who are, by some mischance, buried alive and who wake up in the middle of the night with five or six feet of earth on top of them.

REFERENCES

Chapey, R. (ed.) (1981) *Language intervention strategies in adult aphasia.* Williams & Wilkins, Baltimore

Code, C. and Muller, D.J. (eds) (1983) *Aphasia therapy.* Arnold, London and Baltimore

Davis, G.A. (1980) A critical look at PACE therapy. In R.H. Brookshire (ed.), *Clinical aphasiology proceedings.* BRK, Minneapolis

Geschwind, N. (1965) Disconnection syndromes in animals and man. *Brain, 88,* 585–644

Hodkinson, H.N., Stevens, S.J. and Kenny, R.A. (1984) Is dysphasia a feature of speech in senile dementia of Alzheimer's type? *Journal of Clinical and Experimental Gerontology, 6(3),* 261–7

Holland, A.L. (1982) Observing functional communication of aphasic patients. *Journal of Hearing and Speech Disorders, 47,* 50–6

Katz, R.C. (1986) *Aphasia treatment and microcomputers.* Taylor & Francis, Basingstoke

Miller, N.E. (1981) The nature of cognitive deficit in senile dementia. In N.E. Miller and G.D. Cohen (eds), *Aging,* vol. 15: *Clinical aspects of Alzheimer's disease and senile dementia.* Raven Press, New York

Morton, J. (1985) Naming. In S. Newman and R. Epstein (eds), *Current perspective in dysphasia.* Churchill Livingstone, Edinburgh

Sapir, S. and Aronson, A. (1985) Aphonia after closed head injury. *British Journal of Disorders of Communication, 20,* 229–36

Skinner, C., Wirz, S., Thompson, I. and Davidson, J. (1984) *The Edinburgh Functional Communication Profile.* Winslow Press, Bicester

Thompson, I.M. (1986) *Language pathology in Alzheimer type dementia and associated disorders.* PhD thesis, Edinburgh

Walker, S. (1982) *Investigation of the communication of elderly subjects.* M.Phil. thesis, Sheffield

FURTHER READING

Beasley, B. and Davis, A. (eds) (1981) *Ageing: communication processes and disorders,* Grune & Stratton, New York

Edwards, M. (ed.) (1982) *Communication changes in elderly people.* College of Speech Therapists, London

Gravell, R. (1988) *Communication problems in elderly people.* Croom Helm, London

Obler, L. and Albert, M.L. (eds) (1980) *Language and communication in the elderly.* Lexington Books, Lexington, Massachusetts

Ulatowska, H.K. (ed.) (1985) *The aging brain: communication in the elderly.* Taylor & Francis, London/College Hill Press, San Diego

6

Head Injury and Older People

Una Holden

It is only within recent years that psychologists and other disciplines have begun to ask questions, examine myths and search for answers to the natural progress, as well as to the problems that can be encountered with the process of ageing. One area which remains almost untouched is that of head injury (HI), its effects, outcome and possible treatment or management. Gerontology is a new science, and many aspects are still under-researched. It is only within the past five to six years that serious attempts have been made to examine the various aspects of HI with children, but very few studies include clients over 60 years of age. There is a crying need for more investigations to clarify the assumptions, vagueness and lack of treatment guidelines which are the rule for this age group.

EPIDEMIOLOGY

Overall figures are supplied by epidemiological studies and reports, but apart from delineating mortality rates and the causes of the injury there is a paucity of detail on the nature and severity of the damage. Field (1976) published a useful account of figures for England and Wales for 1972. He indicated an incidence rate of 430/100,000, which was probably over-inclusive. However, this and most of the reports from the USA, though they covered a variety of causes of HI, lacked confirmation of brain damage and provided little to clarify the actual cause of death, possible later complications or the degree and nature of disability sustained by survivors. Furthermore most of these studies are out of date. The 1980 report of the US National Head and Spinal Cord Injury Survey (Anderson,

Kalsbeck and Hartwell, 1980) though indicating an incidence rate of 200/100,000, based on hospital admissions did not include immediate deaths or dead-on-arrival figures.

Most of the earlier reports made consistent reference to the increase of mortality rates with age. Kerr, Kay and Lassman (1971) showed a significant correlation of death with age regardless of the severity of the injury. Carlsonn, van Essen and Lofren (1968) stressed that death due to complications was notable with older patients (1976), while confirming the increase of fatality with age, noted that the peak for the 15–24-year-olds was actually higher and associated with road traffic accidents (RTA) in particular. Falls were particularly high with older people, and those over 65 involved with RTAs were usually pedestrians. All reports indicate an across-age higher incidence rate for men, with one exception — women over 75 have the higher rate, but this could be reflecting the larger number of women surviving into extreme old age.

Several recent studies are providing more useful information. In Scotland Jennett and his colleagues have collected data over the past ten years on a defined population, and have published invaluable statistics (Jennett, Murray, MacMillan, MacFarlane, Bentley and Hawthorne, 1977; Jennett, Murray, Carlin, McKean, MacMillan and Strang, 1979; Jennett and MacMillan 1981). More recently they have focused on the elderly (Jennett, 1982, 1987). Other studies, also on a defined population, are being made available by Kraus, Black, Hessol, Ley, Rokaw, Sullivan, Bowyers, Knowlton and Marshall (1984) in the USA. National figures for England and Wales (OPCS, 1986) are outlined in Table 6.1. These basic figures only provide some indication of the type of injury to which the elderly are prone. They also show that they are only involved in less than a quarter of all traffic accident fatalities, but older women account for nearly all the deaths due to falls.

Jennett (1982) indicates that approximately 1 million HI cases attend British casualty units each year, but only one in five are admitted. Within 48 hours two-thirds are discharged, and about 5 per cent are sent to a neurosurgical unit. In Scotland 830/100,000 patients over 64 years old attend accident clinics in comparison to 1184/100,000 aged 25–64 years.

Admissions: 30 per cent older group, 20 per cent younger group.

Table 6.1: Accident statistics, 1983–5

	1983, all ages	1984, all ages	1985, all ages	1984			1985		
				15–24 years	65–74	75+	15–24 years	65–74	75+
RTA									
Male	3552	3547	3379	1264	227	325	1179	276	323
Female	1507	1465	1453	289	240	353	291	222	362
Falls									
Male	1481	1416	1430	55	238	693	55	231	723
Female	2608	2512	2477	12	264	2074	2	266	2045

Attending casualty: 6 per cent are 64+.

Admission from casuality: 9 per cent are 64+.

Coma longer than 6 hours: 11 per cent are elderly admissions.

Fatalities: 25 per cent are 64+.

Neurosurgical interventions for intracranial haematoma: 13 per cent are 64+.

The figures for Scotland confirm the peaks for highest incidence, mortality and severe brain damage are for the 15–24-year-old group, but Jennett (1982) shows that, despite this, the number of people over 64 years who survive after severe HI is very low indeed. When involved in RTAs the over-64s are more likely to be pedestrians or passengers, and the high rate of falls is often related to alcohol consumption (Field, 1976; Jennett, 1987).

Jennett and MacMillan (1981) provide some interesting comparisons with figures gathered from defined populations in Scotland, England, Wales and the USA. Although not specifically focusing on the elderly the patterns are remarkably similar. Although actual numbers vary a little from year to year the peaks and troughs of the graphs remain much the same even in recent surveys. In comparing figures from the different areas it would seem that the mortality rate is higher in the USA, and the admission rate lower. Also attendance at casualty units is higher than in Britain.

One of the survey areas in the USA mentioned above was San Diego, which in 1980 had a population of 1,861,846 and an incidence of 180/100,000 population rate for brain injury. The study by Kraus *et al.* (1984) provides a detailed account of brain injury in a defined population and a confirmed diagnosis of brain injury, its degree of severity and the outcome, giving equal importance to mortality, admission and discharge rates. This detailed account throws light on the effects on all age groups, but unfortunately does not give age-related details once the consideration of outcome is reached. As in Great Britain, the San Diego mortality and severity peaks occur at the 15–24-year level and rise again after 70 years with the rates for men higher than for women. With regard to falls the rates were approximately 100/100,000 for women and 75/100,000 for men, rising as dramatically as in Great Britain as age increased.

Kraus *et al.* carefully defined brain injury and excluded all cases where this could not be confirmed. All their rates were based on brain injury rather than the broader term Head Injury.

The incidence of brain injury was 180 per 100,000 population
Mortality rate   30 per 100,000 population
Immediate death   21 per 100,000 population
Male brain injury accounted for 70 per cent of all cases.
Incidence of brain injury with reference to age shows peaks:
    15–24 years, 70+ for men.
    0–5 years, 12–24 years, 70+ for women, but the numbers
    are much lower.

Mortality rates in reference to age once again showed the two peaks at 15–24 years and 70+ years for men, the latter being particularly high. Rates for women followed the same pattern but were much lower, particularly for the 70+ age group.

Falls causing brain injury were also higher for men, and two peaks were found at 0–5 years and 65+ years, though over 65 more women sustained injury from falls. The mortality rates were not included here, so a direct comparison with British figures is not possible. RTAs accounted, as in Great Britain, for most brain injuries. Although specific causes of such injury were examined there is no indication of the relationships of such causes to mortality. It is interesting to note that, unlike Britain, the rate of injury to older pedestrians is not particularly high, and the major peaks for RTAs only occur amongst the 15–25-year group. This probably reflects national differences in living. The pedestrian is probably more common in Britain, where fewer old people have the use of a car. Another national difference is reflected in the fact that brain injury due to firearms was highest for men over the age of 65 years in the USA.

Kraus *et al.* provide information on discharge and on outcome, but unfortunately do not relate this to age. Though 83 per cent of patients were discharged home requiring no further care it would be of value to know how many of these were over 65 years and how many of the 2.6 per cent in a special treatment centre belonged to the older group. Further information about recovery rates and levels would prove valuable, and it is to be hoped that a later paper from this centre will provide such information.

Death from complications has been an accepted picture for the over-65s. Carlsonn *et al.* (1968) found a clear distinction between death due primarily to injury sustained in the accident when death occurred within the first 48 hours and mortality due to complications which arose 4–22 days later. Though all ages would be included in the former, complications were almost exclusively found among the older group.

Older people in coma for over six hours are unlikely to regain full independence. Jennett (1987) reports a study with 134 patients over 65 and in coma for over six hours where only 5 per cent regained independent living. The older patient developing an acute intracranial haematoma appears only to benefit from surgery and evacuation if the coma is not deep and if his or her physical state is reasonably good. In such instances the recovery rate is about a quarter, if the coma is deep and the physical state poor the prognosis is not promising.

OTHER RESEARCH FINDINGS

Here too there is a paucity of information and a considerable number of assumptions.

Delayed response to treatment and slow recovery are generally reported. Gronwell and Wrightson (1974) and other investigators examined processing of incoming information and showed that performance returned to normal according to the length of post-traumatic amnesia (PTA); with older people the process took even longer. Persistent memory loss is also related to PTA and age. In many studies vague statements such as 'age appears to be significant' are not helpful, or particularly meaningful. It is said that post-traumatic symptoms are more numerous with older people even when there was no pre-existing emotional or personality disorder. This is taken to imply that the elderly do not adjust well to trauma, or as easily as younger people. Without controlled studies this remains yet another assumption.

Age and recovery from trauma are subject to many such unproven conclusions and variables are ignored. Miller (1984) examines this situation carefully and points out that it is difficult to be sure that comparable damage has occurred to younger and older brains. Different pathology is found, so it is well nigh impossible to find well-matched lesions. Pre-existing experience and behavioural patterns will be different. In children learning of verbal material is very new, so it could be easier to switch to use of the right hemisphere, whereas in adults with a well-established language system a lesion in the left hemisphere will almost certainly have a different outcome. Past experiences, depending on the individual, can help or hinder recovery. Older people may well have some pre-traumatic disease process in operation. There are also external factors which can make a difference to an older person's response to treatment. Attitudes of staff and relatives who have been led to believe that older people's potential for recovery is poor may not provide the attention or assist re-motivation as adroitly as they do with younger people. Other factors, such as the belief that 'You can't teach an old dog new tricks' may influence confidence in attempting retraining and rehabilitative approaches. The general acceptance of such myths leads employers to hesitate to employ older people, so re-employment of an older person post-traumatically becomes even more unlikely. Personal expectations are obviously coloured by the ideas accepted by society, and it is possible that feelings of hopelessness and worthlessness can play a major role in recovery at all ages, but more profoundly in old age.

The work that has been done on age and recovery is far from complete, and the many accepted notions require much more careful investigation. Miller provides, in the same book, an interesting review of animal studies on brain function relating to age. As with other reviews the resultant impression is that such research has failed to clarify very much about head injury and the ageing process.

In the study of human subjects speculation and myth have failed to take several variables into account. Satz and Fletcher (1981) also question the animal–human comparison, stating that the boundaries between human and animal models are indistinct and, furthermore, that the stress laid upon chronological age in relation to plasticity is unwarranted. For instance, it is accepted that an immature brain will recover function more easily than an older one. Contrasting opinions on the recovery rate of the immature brain are rarely cited. Isaacson (1975) refers to this belief in recovery from damage in early youth as another myth, and stresses that evaluation of such damage must include a consideration of transient changes in brain function caused, for example, by diaschisis and the multiple changes that occur — tissue damage, type and degree of damage, its location and the nature of the environment in which it takes place. The last of these is of extreme importance in rates and degrees of recovery at any age. Too frequently it is forgotten that injury at birth and during infancy can result in cerebral palsy and mental retardation. Language is the main source of controversy in the arguments about plasticity, the brain and recovery. Many reports claim that children with left hemisphere damage have learned to use language again when the right hemisphere has become responsible for that function. This is now questioned in the light of recent work. Dennis (1980), using more careful assessments, suggests that this is not completely true. Although spontaneous recovery is possible it is not the rule (Satz and Bullard-Bates, 1981) and equally there is evidence that up to 50 per cent of cases have shown no improvement within a year (Satz and Fletcher, 1981). As stated by several researchers, age is not the only variable to take into account when considering recovery. Lesion size, location, type and acuteness are at least some of the other factors. Satz and Fletcher identify other myths. The risk of aphasia in right-handed adults and children after left hemisphere damage is about the same, and aphasia is more likely to occur following left rather than right hemisphere damage, regardless of age after infancy. The risk of aphasia after right hemisphere damage is rare for all ages after infancy too. Variability in effect of damage is as great in children as in adults. Individual differences occur in all age groups with regard to all language deficits — reading, writing and speech.

Reviewers in general agree that relevant assessment methods may well be missing from many of the reported studies, and are probably missing in clinical practice as well. Until recently measures of intelligence and brain function were limited, and even now leave a great deal to be desired. This has resulted not only in overlooking residual damage but equally many of the signs of improvement are missed.

St James-Roberts (1979) offers two explanations of recovery:

1. Real damage to the central nervous system has not taken place. The effects were transitory and due either to diaschisis or delay in maturation.
2. Recovered behaviour is due to the effects of remaining systems and the additional effects of normal learning.

This brings into focus the theories of brain function over which argument have raged for years (Luria, 1963; Blundell, 1975; Hecaen and Albert, 1975; Miller, 1984) and are closely related to plasticity of the brain. These references should be consulted for further details of the theories which are mentioned only briefly here.

Von Monakow's theory of *diaschisis* links damage to a more or less temporary shock to parts of the brain which are connected in some way to the actual area of damage or lesion. This shock effect is nothing to do with oedema, which is a common occurrence in brain injury. Another theory of brain function is that of *inhibition.* Luria believed that a lesion could stun or disrupt the activity in other parts of the brain, perhaps via interference in neurotransmitter production. The involvement or takeover by *secondary systems* is another possibility. When the original system has recovered, or the parts that are spared can operate effectively, the original system comes into use again. *Reorganisation* implies that another system altogether can become responsible for a damaged function. *Functional adaptation* refers to how a person with brain damage learns to use other ways than those employed previously, to achieve his or her intentions, complete a task or perform an action.

There are many theories on how recovery might be possible, but despite many impressive arguments there is no certainty about any of them.

EFFECTS OF HEAD INJURY

Local injury

Wounds, lacerations, bruises or localised HI may look very unpleasant and appear serious, but open HI is rarely as traumatic in the long term as closed HI, where there may be no external evidence whatsoever. Penetrating wounds due to falls, physical attacks or work accidents usually only involve areas in the immediate vicinity of the wound, there is rarely a contra-coup effect (opposite poles) and fractured bones act as buffers. There may be a resultant limb weakness, a fit or other localised reaction, but loss of consciousness for longer than five minutes is rare, and may not even occur at all. As with any HI careful investigation and follow-up are necessary to ensure that more serious damage to the brain has not occurred.

Closed head injury

Loss of consciousness is of great importance in diagnosis, prognosis and treatment. A period of unconsciousness that exceeds five minutes in duration will almost certainly imply the existence of brain injury, some of which could be permanent. Even mild damage can lead to fatalities. Secondary events can develop after a patient has regained consciousness and apparently talked sensibly to staff and relatives. One-third of HI cases of a fatal nature have suffered from a secondary infection or raised intracranial pressure. Vascular complications also play a major role in fatal outcome.

The effects of HI depend on the direction of the blow, the force and the velocity and the freedom of movement of the head. The site of impact will have contusions and lacerations, and there are also contra-coup effects. If the head is at rest the injuries will be at their maximum at the site of injury. If the head is in motion the contra-coup effects are usually worse.

Acceleration–deceleration. These injuries are the result of movement, force and velocity related to impact. For instance, a motorcyclist may hit another vehicle, be flung into the air and crash either into the vehicle, a wall or the ground. The brain may appear to be well protected lying inside layers of bone, membrane and fluid, but it remains free to move about. With the unfortunate motorcyclist the rate of movement and the force of impact would send the brain crashing about inside the skull. When the rate of movement is considerably accelerated the protective coverings are not sufficient and the brain becomes vulnerable to at the least bruising, and at the worst gross damage. In acceleration–deceleration situations swirling movements in the tissues are caused. These rotational and linear stresses tear up nerve fibres in any part of the brain and damage can be widespread.

Complications

Cerebral oedema. This is swelling which occurs usually around the site of the lesion, and is quite common. As the lesions heal it will settle down, but it can be severe enough to cause infarcts or haematomas, which may lead to death.

Vascular lesions. Little haemorrhages can result from the shearing of nerve fibres and from general injuries. Large and small infarcts may occur and even arteries can become necrotic. Subdural haematomas, blood in the central nervous system and obstructions caused by blood — which leads to a hydrocephalus — are all possible complications of HI.

Cerebral anoxia. Lack of oxygen caused by circulatory disorders, blood loss or breathing problems due to chest injuries can add to the problems of the damaged brain.

Acute stages of HI

1. Impairments of consciousness — from a moment to a prolonged coma.
2. A variable period of confusion and awareness.
3. A variable period of amnesias — PTA (post-traumatic amnesia), RA (retrograde amnesia).

These three stages usually follow on from each other during a course of recovery.

1. Concussion. This results from a blow to the head, or impact with a blunt object. There is a consequent impairment of neuronal function. Loss of consciousness is the obvious feature of this stage. Mild confusion may not indicate permanent effects on the brain, but it is now generally accepted that loss of consciousness for over five minutes indicates that some form of permanent damage will be present. It is also recognised that repeated injury to the head, even over a long period of time, can cause permanent damage.

It can be argued that boxers and other sportspeople can suffer concussion without loss of consciousness. A series of blows to the head, a bad fall or a collision with another player can result in confused thought processes and lethargy over varying periods of time. A boxer who regularly engages in fights can become 'punch-drunk', each damaging bout adding yet more injury to those already sustained. Cumulative effects can be as serious as instant ones.

Minor accidents, as for instance those in sports, should be treated with some caution as delayed effects might occur. The classical example is that of the footballer who, after a collision, loses consciousness for a few seconds, recovers and continues to play — yet later has no recall for any of the events following the collision. Other 'side-effects' such as slurred or confused speech, disorders of perception or movement can appear some time after the trauma, and can reappear from time to time later on.

2. Variable period of awareness. This period between trauma and return to full consciousness and awareness of day-to-day events can be seen in many forms from apparently psychotic behaviour to apathy and withdrawal. It is sometimes referred to as the psychiatric phase. The person may be manic, and staff will be in despair as he or she makes demands, disrupts routines, interferes with others and cannot keep still. Paranoia is possible. The patient may insist that the nurse or doctor was the cause of the accident, and may even become violent. Thinking is often confabulated, learning is impaired and confused. Hallucinations and delusions are quite common, so is disorientation for time, place and person.

On the other hand the person may appear quite sensible most of the time, and staff and relatives are given the impression that he or she has returned to normal.

With elderly people this period can be severe and extended. It may persist for months, and observers conclude that a dementia is present. A poor physical state, a history of alcoholism or vascular disorders can extend this phase of recovery.

3. Particular amnesic effects. (a) Post-traumatic amnesia (PTA) plays an important role in judging the degree of severity of an injury and the prognosis. PTA refers to the period of time from the moment of the accident and loss of consciousness to the time when the person becomes continuously aware of events around him or her and is capable, once again, of remembering day-to-day happenings. As apparent clarity of thought and speech can occur during PTA it is often difficult to be sure when the PTA is over. Patients can usually confirm this themselves.

Some of the periods of lucidity can be recalled later, but generally the entire period after the accident has not been stored in a retrievable manner, and that time and the events have been completely lost. The length of PTA is very important, as the longer it is the more severe the brain damage. The accepted rule is:

0–5 minutes	mild concussion
less than 1 hour	mild deficits
1–24 hours	moderate deficits
1–7 days	severe deficits
more than 7 days	very severe deficits.

PTA has implication for return to work (Steadman and Graham, 1970).

PTA less than an hour	1 month
PTA less than a day	2 months
PTA less than a week	4 months
PTA more than a week	at least a year, if at all.

Studies are also suggesting a link with social recovery, and with the development of psychiatric sequelae.

With elderly people memory may remain unsteady even after a lengthy PTA.

(b) Retrograde amnesia (RA) is the time between the moment of injury and loss of consciousness to the last clear, continuous memory *before* the accident. This is usually shorter than PTA but not always so. It is normally only for a few minutes, and the person can even remember leaving home or other events shortly before the incident. Mild cases may have no RA at all. In serious cases RA may encompass days, weeks, or even months. Often as the patient recovers the RA period becomes shorter and shorter as more memories return. Sometimes RA actually lengthens. It is extremely rare for the patient with anything more than a moderate concussion to remember the actual accident.

The unusually long RAs are often thought to be psychogenic, but there is evidence that they can also be organic. Very little research has been completed on RA, and it would be interesting to know how often elderly people suffer from an extended RA in comparison with younger patients. PTA and RA have been rather loosely left to the injured person's judgement — usually quite satisfactorily. The Galveston Orientation and Amnesia Test (GOAT) developed by Levin, Grossman, Rose and Teasdale (1979) can be used as a more objective assessment of both PTA and RA periods.

More detailed accounts of HI, its diagnosis, prognosis and treatment can be found in textbooks such as Strub and Black (1981) and Jennett and Teasdale (1981).

Other complications

It is important not to miss evidence of fracture, epilepsy, meningitis and haematoma. About 5 per cent, or approximately 5000 patients per year, will have a fit within seven days. This may prove a problem in the future as epileptic fits can reoccur up to four years later. The degree and risk of epilepsy can now be estimated fairly accurately.

Even after consciousness and awareness have been regained brain damage can be so severe as to cause permanent damage to abilities and daily living skills. Handicaps are often physical — broken bones which fail to recover full mobility for the person, disfiguring scars, etc., but there are also permanent or persistent impairments to brain function. During at least the following two years post-trauma, improvements occur, but changes will result in work and social outlets. Aphasias and physical disabilities are expected, but other more subtle changes can cause friction at home, at work and socially. The effects on personality, memory and intellectual ability are harder to accept and understand.

Many patients over 64 years of age develop a chronic subdural haematoma and this is frequently overlooked as there is no record of an HI. Its identification depends on general practitioners, geriatricians and psychiatrists who have noticed the presence of persistent headaches and slight weakness or paralysis. The patient will probably show evidence of recent deterioration in intellectual abilities. Surgical interventions are usually quite successful. On the other hand, acute intracranial haematomas which occur within the first few days or week post-trauma are less promising prognostically with older people.

ASSESSMENT PROCEDURES

Assessing the degree and severity of HI covers a wide range. Obviously, CAT scans, radiography and laboratory investigations are of particular importance. Here, more observational assessments will be considered. The scale which is probably most widely used is the Glasgow Coma Scale (Jennett and Teasdale, 1981). This simple instrument concentrates on the opening of eyes and the quality of verbal and motor responses. Staff can monitor reactions during the first few hours or days after injury, and by carefully recording response or lack of response can judge changes in the patient's conscious condition.

The Glasgow Outcome Scale (Jennett and Teasdale, 1981) has five categories which simply state degrees of disablement from persistent vegetative state to full recovery, which is used over a period of six months as a guide to prognosis.

The Rancho Los Amigos Scale of Cognitive Levels and Expected Behaviour (Hagen and Malkmus, 1979) looks at behavioural stages in the progress of recovery and concentrates on the highest level of cognitive functioning that is present throughout the recovery period.

At a later stage, after PTA, other neuropsychological investigations might be introduced. Obviously these will be presented in keeping with the individual's ability to respond or to concentrate. The elderly, in particular, will require gentle approaches (see Chapter 2).

It is advisable with older people to beware of assumptions regarding laterality. Just because everyone believes that he or she is right-handed, or because he or she always writes with the right hand, it still does not follow that the person really is left hemisphere dominant. Until recent years left-handed children were persuaded, or even forced, to write with the traditional right hand. Left-handedness was regarded as socially unacceptable or something to joke about, so teachers and often parents stressed the 'proper' use of the right hand. This enforced change can lead to problems and errors in assessment and location of damage. A 'right'-handed person might have brain damage which is being overlooked because there is no language disorder. Equally such a person who can also write with the left hand may have language problems instead of perceptual or spatial difficulties, that are not noticed. If the person is unable to communicate he or she cannot explain the ambidexterity. Without careful questioning and close observation this 'crossed' laterality could lead to errors in the identification of impairments, and limit the degree of useful assistance available to the patient.

EFFECTS OF HEAD INJURY ON ELDERLY PEOPLE

Most studies and papers on HI pay scant attention to the special problems of older people. They imply that it has a devastating effect even on healthy and active old people. It is reported that they take longer to recover than younger patients, longer to regain interests and abilities, longer to regain awareness, continue to have memory problems even after PTA has passed, remain in hospital longer and have a higher mortality rate. Survivors deteriorate dramatically, and the prognosis for independent living is poor.

This negative and dismissive account is reminiscent of another 'attitude' regarding old people — the belief that age and dementia are synonymous, and that the label 'dementia' implies that 'nothing can be done'. As the statements are based on untested, anecdotal and uncontrolled situations they cannot be accepted as fact. It is not logical to assume that nothing can be done when nothing is being done. Before accepting that deterioration will usually accompany HI in elderly people some form of intervention, some changes in care and retraining programmes should be introduced in a controlled study and proper comparisons made. Little has been done to define problems more clearly, to provide realistic goals or appropriate retraining programmes. There appears to have been no attempt to consider the effects of the environment — both physical and psychological — on head-injured elderly people. Support systems should be checked.

Younger patients have family and friends who are anxious and able to help, and this is recognised as a major factor in recovery (Satz and Fletcher, 1981; Miller, 1984). It is highly probable that psychological factors are of relevance in the recovery of older people as well. The person may well live alone, lack loving support and have nothing worthwhile to which he or she can return. The prospect of coping with daily living and self-care in a disabled state can severely affect motivation and the will to live. The prospect of survival in a lonely, unfriendly world is not one that would convince an older person — or anyone else for that matter — that it is worth the effort. The reality is that such a person would require some form of long-term institutional care, and dependency would be high. Such a future is not one that would be eagerly embraced by many. However, most individuals do wish to live, their disabilities and motivation require attention and more support should be made available to them. In practice no effort, or very little, is made to provide suitable programmes or to consider relevant approaches to the problems of recovery and rehabilitation for the older generation.

Not only are rehabilitation and resettlement schemes of importance, but the actual quality of care for old people should be examined. Physical and neurological care is undoubtedly of a high standard, but the understanding of psychological and environmental factors remains poor. The attitudes towards, and beliefs about, age continue unchallenged, and this aspect is omitted in staff training. Until the special needs, strengths and particular problems of the over-65s with HI are taken into serious consideration most of the statements about HI and age remain dubious and probably based on false premises.

Certain centres in a number of countries offer a team approach to the problems faced by those with HI and their families. Unfortunately not all such victims are so fortunate, and the service that they are offered leaves much to be desired. The lack of knowledge and understanding of age increases the likelihood that the elderly will receive limited care and inappropriate treatment.

TWO CASE REPORTS

A brief account of two cases where HI was suspected in older people might serve to demonstrate how easy it is for staff or the general public to make assumptions without logical enquiry.

Case 1

Mr S was brought into a general hospital ward after falling in the street and losing consciousness. He was confused for some time after. Three days later the staff reported that he was still confused, disorientated and apparently deteriorating mentally. A scan was booked, but radiography had provided no evidence of a fracture. As he had been drinking prior to the fall it was suspected that he might be an alcoholic.

While awaiting the scan the neuropsychologist was asked for an opinion.

Mr S was about 75 years of age and lived alone, was active, independent and had plenty of friends. The staff were particularly concerned about his ability to continue to care for himself. After a general discussion Mr S explained that he could not remember exactly what happened to him. He suspected that he had had 'one too many' when he went for his regular Sunday lunchtime visit to the pub. When asked simple questions relating to time and place his response was that he had no idea. When gently pressed to provide more information he replied, 'If you look out the windows here what can you see? Nothing but blank walls. There is no clock, no newspaper and no-one to talk to. I was 'out cold' when I came here and I don't know how long that lasted. No-one has told me a thing and I've no means of finding out the answers to any of your questions.'

When told the name of the hospital he accurately described its whereabouts. He was informed of his length of stay, and told the day and date. The following day he had no difficulty in responding to any orientation questions recalling the events around his admission as explained the previous day, and his general response was normal. No evidence was found to support the assumption that he was other than naturally confused after his fall. Within a couple of days he was discharged home perfectly fit and able.

Here the problem lay with the environment and with staff assumptions, rather than with the patient or the sustained injuries. Simple common sense and a more informative environment would have avoided unnecessary stress for Mr S and made the problem easier to solve.

Case 2

Miss K, aged 87 years, had been knocked down by a car six months prior to neuropsychological investigations. She had sustained some physical injuries and walked with a slight limp. Her lawyer was seeking compensation for injury, but felt that at such an age she could only be demonstrating some degree of 'senility', and it would be impossible to differentiate this from any brain damage in a way which would convince a court of law.

Miss K had been a student of Carl Jung, and had eventually specialised in treating childhood disorders. Although she had only retired two years previously she was still toying with the idea of opening another treatment centre. She felt that, possibly, this might be unrealistic in view of her age! On examination it was quickly established that she was of very superior intelligence and a highly cultured woman. She proved to be rather garrulous, but her performance on neuropsychological and other tests was almost perfect.

Three months before her accident, when she was 86 years old, she had been in Denmark where she travelled about the country on a hired moped! This remarkable woman had no knowledge of the Danish language but had found it no problem to follow the International road signs. Three months prior to the accident she was perfectly capable of interpreting visual material; on testing six months after the accident she had great difficulty in interpreting any material of a similar nature.

The court awarded damages which made her remaining years, spent in a private and comfortable residential home, very comfortable.

In the case of Miss K it was assumed that because of her age it would be impossible to differentiate between impairments caused by injury and those which could be attributed to 'normal' decline.

Suggestions regarding rehabilitation

While it is vital that appropriate investigations and treatment for HI should be instigated as soon as possible, it is also important that a team approach should be employed, as far as possible, with the elderly as well as with any other age group. Consideration should be given to the following:

1. Medical and neurological investigations and procedures.
2. A good assessment of social background and influences.
3. At the appropriate time in recovery assessments should be made by the relevant disciplines — speech therapy, physiotherapy, neuropsychology, occupational therapy, etc.
4. Observations by nursing staff should be carefully recorded.
5. Team discussion and suitable management and treatment programmes should be initiated as soon as possible. Goal-setting should be made with care.
6. The environment should be modified to suit the patient.
7. Monitoring should be continual in the early stages, and regular later on.
8. Consideration should be given to useful and meaningful ways to motivate the patient and give encouragement.
9. Provision of a meaningful support system. The spouse, if living, might be frail, or the person might be living in isolation.

At the stage in which awareness is only transient, and PTA still in operation, a simple form of reality orientation can be of assistance (Corrigan, Arnett, Houck and Jackson, 1985; Holden and Woods, 1982/8), not only to the elderly but all recovering from trauma or a coma state. Simple procedures such as a stable environment, familiar faces and common-sense aids to regaining body image are invaluable. The person's knowledge and interests are important tools in achieving awareness of the self. Each contact with the person regaining consciousness should provide an opportunity for reorientation.

Personal identity and orientation can be re-established by using a patient's own hand to feel his or her hot forehead, accompanied by a statement such as 'Do you feel hot; there, can you feel your forehead, does it feel hot?' and 'Would you like to wash your face? Here's a face cloth, now you try to wash, it may make you feel better'. A guiding hand can help the patient to begin again to associate sensation with self-awareness. The use of 'Get well' cards signed by family and friends can be the start of rehabilitation, which will accelerate if such information is provided on a regular basis, encouraging recognition, the use of basic skills and memory. This early contact is also a means of letting the person know that someone cares, that there is a reason to recover, and implants a sense of worth with which motivation is fed.

This kind of programme is valuable to young people, but it is every bit as important to the old who need warmth and prompting in order to motivate and reassure them. Without such early and continued support it is hardly surprising that they deteriorate or remain withdrawn for a longer period than the young.

Proper assessments will provide clues as to the areas of damage and retained ability. More structured rehabilitation programmes with this in mind should be initiated as soon as the person is physically and emotionally ready. If the process of establishing good relationships and encouraging progress has been in operation since the first signs of minimal awareness then such programmes can develop smoothly and easily. They will also have a better chance of success and provide more opportunities to estimate the validity of the so far accepted belief that older people have a poorer prognosis post-trauma than younger people.

REFERENCES

Anderson, D.W., Kalsbeck, W.D. and Hartwell, T.D. (1980) The national head and spinal cord survey: design and methodology. *Journal of Neurosurgery, 53,* 811–18

Blundell, J. (1975) *Physiological psychology.* Essential Psychology Series. Methuen, London

Carlsonn, C.A., van Essen, C. and Lofren, J. (1968) Factors affecting the clinical course of patients with severe head injuries. Parts 1 and 2. *Journal of Neurosurgery, 29,* 242–51

Corrigan, J.D., Arnett, J.A., Houck, L.J. and Jackson, R.D. (1985) Reality orientation for brain injured patients: group treatment and monitoring of recovery. *Archives of Physical Medicine and Rehabilitation, 66,* 626–39

Dennis, M. (1980) Strokes in childhood. 1: Communication, intent, expression and comprehension after left hemisphere arteriopathy in a right handed nine year old. In R.W. Reiber (ed.), *Language, development and aphasia in children.* Academic Press, New York

Field, J.H. (1976) *Epidemiology of head injuries in England and Wales.* Her Majesty's Stationery Office, London

Gronwell, D. and Wrightson, P. (1974) Delayed recovery of intellectual function after minor head injury. *Lancet, ii,* 605–9

Hagen, C. and Malkmus, D. (1979) *Intervention strategies for language disorders secondary to head trauma.* American Speech–Language–Hearing Association Short Courses, Atlanta

Hecaen, H. and Albert, M.L. (1975) *Human neuropsychology.* Wiley, New York

Holden, U.P. and Woods, R.T. (1982/8) *Reality orientation,* 2nd edn. Churchill Livingstone, Edinburgh and New York

Isaacson, R.L. (1975) The myth of recovery from early brain damage. In N.G. Ellis (ed.), *Aberrant development in infancy.* Wiley, New York

Jennett, B. (1982) 'Head Injury in the elderly'. In F.I. Caird (ed.), *Neurosurgical disorders in the elderly.* Wright, Bristol

Jennett, B. (1987) 'Head injuries in the older patient'. (In press)

Jennett, B. and MacMillan, R. (1981) Epidemiology of head injury. *British Medical Journal, 282,* 101–4

Jennett, B. and Teasdale, G. (1981) *Management of head injuries.* F.A. Davies, Philadelphia

Jennett, B., Murray, A., MacMillan, R., MacFarlane, J., Bentley, C. and Hawthorne, V. (1977) Head injuries in Scottish hospitals. *Lancet, ii,* 696–8

Jennett, B., Murray, A., Carlin, J., McKean, M., MacMillan, R. and Strang, I. (1979) Head injuries in three Scottish hospitals. *British Medical Journal, 2,* 955–8

Kerr, T.A., Kay, D.W.K. and Lassman, L.P. (1971) Characteristics of patients, type of accident and mortality in a consecutive series of head injuries admitted to a neurosurgical unit. *British Journal of Preventive and Social Medicine, 25,* 179–85

Kraus, J.P., Black, M.A., Hessol, N., Ley, F., Rokaw, W., Sullivan, C., Bowyers, S., Knowlton, S. and Marshall, L. (1984) The incidence of acute brain injury and serious impairment in a defined population. *American Journal of Epidemiology, 119*(2), 186–201

Levin, H.S., Grossman, R.G., Rose, J.E. and Teasdale, G. (1979) Long term neuropsychological outcome of closed head injury. *Journal of Neurosurgery, 50,* 412–22

Luria, A.R. (1963) *Restoration of function after brain injury.* Pergamon Press, Oxford

Miller, E. (1984) *Recovery and management of neuropsychological impairments.* Wiley, Chichester and New York

Office of Population Censuses and Surveys (1986) *Mortality rates in England and Wales.* OPCS Monitor DH2 86/2

St James-Roberts, I. (1979) Neurological plasticity, recovery from brain insult and child development. In H.W. Reese and L.P. Lipsitt (eds), *Advances in child development and behaviour,* vol. 14. Academic Press, New York, pp. 254–319

Satz, P. and Bullard-Bates, C. (1981) Acquired aphasia in children. In M.T. Sarno (ed.), *Acquired aphasia.* Academic Press, New York

Satz, P. and Fletcher, J.M. (1981) Emergent trends in neuropsychology: an overview. *Journal of Consulting and Clinical Psychology, 49*(6), 851–65

Steadman, J.J. and Graham, J.G. (1970) Head injuries: an analysis and

175

follow-up study. *Proceedings of the Royal Society of Medicine, 63,* 23–8

Strub, R.L. and Black, F.W. (1981) *Organic brain syndromes.* F.A. Davis, Philadelphia

7

Hyperventilation

Una Holden

Departments of clinical psychology and neurology are presented
with many problems that are not always clearly associated with
neuropsychology and yet are appropriately referred to that
specialty. Clinicians are asked to treat such conditions as torti-
collis, writer's cramp, folie-à-deux, functional blindness,
deafness and weakness of limbs, tics, pain and other behavioural
reactions. These are often related to emotional stress, but could
also be responses to physical disorders. People over the age of
60 years are just as likely to be victims of these disorders as
younger adults. One of the commonest 'fringe' disorders
referred to a department of clinical psychology is hyperventilation (HV) and an active neuropsychology unit can be asked to
treat between six and twelve cases a week. A large percentage
of these cases are people over the age of 60 years.

Elderly people present a more complex picture than younger
adults as their anxieties are often hidden or overshadowed by
their physical, or even organic, conditions. It is relevant in a
book on neuropsychology and the elderly to provide a chapter
specifically on the subject of HV as there are essential difficulties in the approach and treatment programmes. It is easy to
overlook, or even to overemphasise HV with the elderly. For
instance, a stroke victim may be in a panic and yet the stroke
problems only are noted. On the other hand, all the gasping,
panting or dizziness may be put down to hysteria and the real
physical or emotional problems which have provoked this
reaction could be overlooked. Elderly HV patients sent to a
neurologist include those with panic attacks, migraine, pain,
epilepsy, vertigo, tremor, paralyses as well as cerebro-vascular
conditions and many other problems.

As HV has only recently become more widely recognised it is

relevant here to provide an outline of its history and the mechanisms involved, before dealing more specifically with its importance in rehabilitation programmes for elderly people.

HISTORY AND BACKGROUND

Until about 1980 the condition was rarely, if ever, considered, and there were no recognised or possible treatment programmes. Awareness of such a disorder was limited to the very few. Even now it is not included in the DSM III Classification of mental disorders. Arguments about the existence of hyperventilation (HV) and various investigations and research have been presented in scientific literature since the beginning of the century (Haldane and Poulton, 1908; Cannon, 1920; Pfeffer, 1978; Lum, 1981; Bass and Gardner, 1985a,b; Kartsounis and Turpin, 1987). The first observer on record appears to be André du Laurens, who in 1559 accurately described such a state. It was he who related it to too much sighing, taking in too much 'ayre' and becoming too emotional. Haldane and Poulton demonstrated it in 1908 to the Physiological Society. Despite this early identification of overbreathing the condition has been ignored by physicians until recent years. Just about every medical specialty and every general practitioner has been faced by an inexplicable set of problems for which there is, apparently, no diagnostic classification or treatment process. As a result the number of neuroses and functional disorders recorded has risen considerably. Details of the general history, causes and effects of HV will not be given here and can be found elsewhere (Lum, 1975; Pfeffer, 1978; Kartsounis, 1987), as this chapter is specifically concerned with the implications of this condition for the elderly. However, a brief outline is relevant.

Breathing is unconscious, but it can be brought into conscious control. The main muscles involved include the diaphragm, the intercostal muscles (those between the ribs) and accessory muscles attached to the outer chest. All of these can be moved under voluntary control and independently of each other. This means that everyone can breathe in a different way. Athletes and opera singers, for instance, need to control their breathing and are taught how to use it to aid their skills. Frequently thoracic forms of breathing become habitual, and when not performing, certain professionals may well continue to breathe from the thorax. Too often when no longer following their profession these people can develop strange and frightening symptoms which they have never previously experienced.

Breathing is a means of getting oxygen into the blood stream and is the principal way of regulating the acid–base balance of the blood. Overbreathing causes too much carbon dioxide to be eliminated from the lungs, thus producing respiratory alkalosis. Hypocarbia (abnormally low level of carbon dioxide in the blood stream) has proved hard to estimate or identify in the past, and this led scientists to dismiss HV as a useless concept (Wood, 1941). However, there are now improved methods of investigation, e.g. an infrared analyser, which have established that HV should be considered as the cause of certain symptoms and is a condition requiring treatment.

Clear diagnosis of HV remains a problem, and full medical investigations are required to rule out other specific explanations for the patient's symptoms. It must be remembered, however, that HV can be present alongside other physical disorders — heart conditions, cancer, metabolic disorders, etc. Voluntary overbreathing (McKell and Sullivan, 1947) or the hyperventilation provocation test (HPT) has been widely used as a diagnostic tool. This requires the patient to breathe in and out very deeply and harshly for one to three minutes. Unusual symptoms will be precipitated even in healthy subjects. In HV individuals the symptoms of which they complain will be provoked very quickly. The period of recovery after such an over-breathing session will vary, and is often considered to be relevant to the diagnosis. Controversy about HPT is based on its subjective nature. Many feel that in order to provide convincing evidence monitoring of physiological changes should be maintained through the HPT (Kartsounis and Turpin, 1987), e.g. heart rate, skin conductance and respiration.

The various effects of physiological processes are responsible for the production of symptoms related to specific changes. For instance, reduction in cerebral oxygenation may cause dizziness and lightheadedness, the lowering of serum-ionized calcium may cause shaking, tremor and tingling sensations and the effect on the autonomic nervous system can result in sweating, chest pain and tightness suggestive of a heart condition. Kartsounis in an excellent, as yet unpublished, review distinguishes seven different categories:

179

1. Neurological (disturbances of consciousness, dizziness, faintness, feelings of unreality, paraesthesia, tingling or coldness of the extremities).
2. Cardiovascular (precordial pain, tachycardia, palpitations).
3. Respiratory (sighing, shortness of breath, tightness of chest).
4. Musculoskeletal (muscle tension, myalgia, tremors, twitches, even tetany).
5. Gastrointestinal (epigastric pain, aerophagy, oral dryness, nausea).
6. Psychological (tension, depersonalisation, free-floating anxiety).
7. Miscellaneous/general (weakness, exhaustion, tinnitus, sleep disturbance, headache).

So clinically a person may present with tingling in the fingers, face or limbs, pins and needles, spots before the eyes, pains, palpitations or flutters, cramps, sick feelings, asthma, epileptiform attacks, panic attacks, heartburn, inability to swallow, migraines, etc. The situation may be that the individual is only mildly affected; on the other hand the disabling effects can be so great that considerable time may be spent on investigations of a wide-ranging nature. Exasperated physicians, unable to find reasonable answers, can add to the patient's distress by informing him or her that the disorder is all in the imagination.

Six to ten per cent of cases referred to the many specialties presenting with such symptoms are hyperventilators. The incidence varies from 3.5 per cent in out-patient clinics to 26 per cent in the specialties. About 10 per cent of the population breathe incorrectly. Many people become lifelong invalids because HV has been overlooked — apparently including Charles Darwin and Florence Nightingale.

There are various theories about the association of HV with personality type — the over-conscientious, perfectionistic person for instance. Whilst athletes and singers are probably perfectionists it would seem more likely that their training is more at fault than their personalities. Alcohol can have interesting though dangerous effects on HV individuals. Drinking and driving for the hyperventilator are more perilous than for those who breathe correctly, as intoxication occurs more speedily. HV plays a part in cults — voodoo, crowd hysteria, satanism and so forth. Even to laugh too hard or cry too much can produce overbreathing, and the ensuing symptoms of HV. It is also said that it is unwise for men to forcibly stick out their chests or for women to mimic Marilyn Monroe!

HYPERVENTILATION AND THE ELDERLY

It is hardly likely that the over-60s would wish to seriously pursue the image of beef-cake or cheese-cake! However, HV is very common and elderly people pay regular calls on their doctors for an explanation of strange and unwelcome symptoms and disorders. Fear of illness plays a large role in the lives of many members of the older generation. Although the majority have no wish to be ill, to be taken as old and fragile, or incapable of living normal lives, there are those who, for various reasons, are looking for support and consideration, and minor complaints can build up if a satisfactory answer is not supplied.

The falls, dizzy spells and the pain reported by some elderly people can be directly associated with HV. These clients can be observed to overbreathe; it is even possible to hear the rate of breathing which can sound like panting or gasping. The individual can become convinced of the existence of lung or heart abnormalities, and his or her gasp breathing will increase not only the rate, but also the degree, of anxiety. While recounting the symptoms in a clinic the increased rate and gasping become pronounced in many cases. Old people in hospital or residential home can also show these signs of distress when threatened or stressed by some problem or concern, and often when confronted with a situation of which they do not approve, or feel unable to change. Although HV should be treated it is just as important to identify the source of possible anxieties or perceived threats, and make necessary modifications in order to minimise anxiety-provoking situations. HV may be only part of the individual's difficulty, and although specific measures can be provided to ease this, other factors may be of equal or even greater importance.

While accepting that HV may well be associated with disease processes, illness and psychiatric disorders, there are many situations provoking HV where anxiety appears to be the main precipitant. Although it is desirable to have clear-cut evidence for a diagnosis of HV it is not always desirable for an elderly person to undergo strenuous, intense investigations. There are other ways to conclude that HV is the most probable cause of problems or additional problems, and ways to develop treatment programmes. These would include:

1. Consider the individual.
2. Using all available information on that individual, examine the various possibilities.
3. Obtain some baseline for the person's level of functioning and ability.
4. Make due allowance for frailty, illness and disability.
5. Provide a programme tailored to that individual's needs.
6. Discuss the plan with the client, staff, physician and relatives.
7. Check to see if stress is caused by changeable or modifiable external influences, e.g. total isolation, mounting bills, unkind staff or relatives, bereavement.
8. Carefully monitor the effects of change, and of treatment.

If a person is breathing at a rate of over 20 breaths a minute, and there is no evidence to associate this overbreathing with a particular physical complaint, it is reasonable to suspect the presence of HV. Even when there is a clear medical diagnosis and HV is also present, proper breathing can prove efficacious in controlling some of the effects of the disease process.

TREATMENT PROGRAMMES

Various programmes for treatment of HV have been provided by physiotherapists and others (Lum, 1977), and research studies have examined the value of such interventions (e.g. Clark, Salkovskis and Chalkley, 1985; Kartsounis, 1987). Work has been done with children and adults, but there are no reports of interventions with the elderly. Here a flexible approach will be outlined which will require modifying to suit the special needs of each individual.

The following explanations and exercises form the basis of any intervention. The inclusion of any of these is at the discretion of the therapist, and not all of them will be relevant to each presenting problem.

Explanation

Discussion of the actual effects of overbreathing is provided. Athletes and singers can be cited as examples of people engaged in activities which demand thoracic breathing, or heavy, deep intakes of breath. It is natural to breathe fast when running, doing something strenuous or even living at high altitudes. The body will adapt to this, but not to periodic or transitory overbreathing bouts. So, although heavier breathing when climbing stairs or carrying things might be normal, the quick or sighing breaths as a general rule are not. If an inward look at breathing is taken at different periods of the day it will be noticed that the rate, depth and nature of breathing does change. Under stress it will speed up. The dangers of taking the traditional 'deep breath' should be discussed as well.

This explanation is important as a preliminary, as clients may take some convincing that their 'serious' symptoms are simply due to overbreathing.

Exercise 1

HPT, as it is a drastic measure for the elderly, should not be used with the majority of old people, but can be used if the client is a young–old person and generally fit and active. If it is used the time must be limited to about 30 seconds and the therapist must keep a careful watch for undue stress.

The client can be reminded of the great, gasping breaths taken by weight-lifters before reaching for the weights. The client is asked to take rasping or gasping breaths, really fiercely, up to the time he or she is told to stop. After a few seconds the complaints should be manifested. A paper bag must be ready. The client is told to breathe into the bag and reinhale the exhaled air in the bag until the symptoms settle down. The bag must cover the nose and mouth completely in order to provide the most efficient aid to recovery.

Such a demonstration can have a profound effect on the client's belief in the therapist's argument!

Exercise 2

A less stressful exercise is more appropriate for elderly people. The client is asked to breathe as normally as possible and at the same time count to himself or herself the number of breaths taken. It is necessary to explain this carefully and several times, as the instructions are often misinterpreted and each part of the breathing process can be counted instead of the required full breath. Each full breath consists of inhalation and exhalation. In other words each 'in' *and* 'out' counts as 'one'. The therapist silently times 60 seconds and then asks 'How many breaths?' Contrary to popular belief 16 breaths to each 60 seconds is too fast. In fact anything over twelve indicates some degree of unsatisfactory breathing process.

Ideally nine or ten breaths a minute should be the pattern of breathing. If the client states any number over 20 the therapist could respond: 'I only took nine. This is the number of breaths you should be taking too, or at least something like that.'

It is advisable to check that the person counted correctly. If so, the idea that another person can take so many fewer breaths is usually sufficiently impressive to encourage cooperation.

Practice methods

The methods provided for the person to use on his or her own are dependent on individual needs and specific difficulties. They can consist of one or more of the following:

Second hand

It is useful if the client has a second hand on a watch or on a clock at home. A large-faced clock with clear numbers and distinctive hands is particularly useful for older people.

It is explained that there are twelve numbers on the clock face and each number also represents five seconds. If the client takes one full breath in each five seconds he or she will be breathing at a rate of twelve breaths in a minute. This may be too fast still, but it is a good guide and usually a reasonable rate for the older generation. To slow the breathing even more, practice at this rate will provide feedback for pacing and then by slightly extending the breaths five breaths in 30 seconds or ten in 60 seconds can be attained. However, the usual problem is that the breathing rate is as much as 24 breaths, or more, a minute, and it is unrealistic to expect the person to make a sudden drop in the rate. Furthermore a target of 12 breaths would seem a more realistic eventual aim. The targets can be staged as follows:

1½ full breaths to each 5 seconds	= 18 in a minute.
8 full breaths to each 30 seconds	= 16 in a minute.
1 full breath to each 5 seconds	= 12 in a minute.
1 full breath in each 6 seconds	= 10 to a minute.

The client is told to 'breathe slowly, easily and shallowly'.

Breathing from the stomach

To help awareness of diaphragmatic breathing instead of the more dangerous chest or thoracic breathing, the client should be encouraged to lie down and to place one hand, or a book, on the stomach. Movement of the hand or book will indicate if breathing is correct and if the right muscles are being used. There should be little or no movement from the chest. As the breath goes out the stomach goes in. As the breath goes in the stomach goes out.

Mental strategy

When the patient has no watch or clock with a second hand, or for some reason — as for example — blindness, cannot see the hands then another strategy can be employed. Mental counting, using 'One thousand, two thousand' can prove helpful as it can be geared to the correct rate. The patient is taught to say slowly to himself or herself 'one thousand' for breathing in, and 'two thousand' for breathing out. The rate can be slowed even further by saying, mentally, 'one thousand, two thousand' whilst inhaling and 'three thousand, four thousand' whilst exhaling. So:

Stage 1: 'One thousand, two thousand. One thousand, two thousand ...'. Where 'one thousand' is for 'in' and two thousand' is for 'out'.

Stage 2: 'One thousand two thousand. Three thousand four thousand. One thousand two thousand. Three thousand four thousand ...'. Where 'one thousand two thousand' is for 'in' and 'three thousand four thousand' is for 'out'. This rate is quite slow and may not be attainable by the more fragile elderly hyperventilators.

Taped exercises

Another strategy, particularly helpful with the elderly, is to provide a tape. Some of the above instructions could be recorded, but the main purpose is to provide timing aids. The therapist will drone:

Innnnnnnnnnn   Ouuuuuuuuuuut ...

to the exact rate of breathing required. Each required rate can be included so that the exercises are staged to reach the individual's target. Each droned 'Innn' and 'Ouuut' staged rate should continue for approximately two to three minutes. If appropriate, the ideal nine to ten rate is also included. Clients find this very helpful, though therapists themselves take some time to develop the drone at the necessary pace. They also need time to overcome an early tendency to giggle!

Another possible taped exercise would be appropriate for the more active and independent elderly. Here a muscle relaxation programme could be offered. It will be necessary to go over this with the client before encouraging practice at home. As these programmes are common to all departments concerned with mental health it is not necessary to outline one here.

General advice

The client could be encouraged to watch for changes in rate throughout the day. He or she could note how stresses change the pattern, and learn how natural it is for the rate to increase under particular conditions such as climbing the stairs or doing something strenuous. The occasions when there does not appear to be any good reason for changes should also be noted.

The old belief that to 'take a deep breath' is useful for stressful situations should also be discussed. It is important to make the client aware of the dangers of taking a deep breath; how, rather than being helpful, it is something to avoid. Sometimes when trying to breathe more slowly gagging occurs, or the person might feel sick. If this should happen then it is helpful to take the deep breath, as long as the breath is *exhaled very slowly*. A couple of swallows can also help.

In learning how to breathe correctly concentrating on breathing can become stressful too. If this should happen then the person should forget all about it for a time. He or she could think of pleasant things, or even do something pleasant. Listening to music, watching an amusing television programme or whatever can induce feelings of peace.

Finally, it is vital to stress that there is nothing strange or odd about the condition. Perfectly normal, healthy and fit people of any age can 'suffer' from HV.

Exercises as outlined above can increase awareness of breathing and the correct way to breathe. They can help anxiety and even lessen difficulties caused by medical, neurological and psychiatric conditions.

CASE STUDIES

Case 1

Mrs A was a lady of 76 years. She had suffered a stroke the previous year which caused both expressive and receptive aphasia. This had proved difficult to treat. To complicate matters she also had dyspraxia and agnosia. She would not respond to instructions regarding movement tasks; nor did she recognise colours or objects when these were only presented visually. Even further complications arose when medical investigations suggested a possible left ventricular failure. The geriatrician was very dubious about the heart condition and suspected an emotionally induced hyperventilation syndrome.

A neuropsychological investigation helped to clarify the issue, but also provided evidence of yet more deficits which could have a profound effect on treatment programmes.

Mrs A did not have real apraxia or agnosia. They appeared to be present because a frontal deficit gave the impression that she could not interpret perceptions accurately or make movements correctly. The aphasia played a major role as it limited her comprehension, but the frontal deficit made her ability to function normally even more difficult. This impairment consisted of severe perseveration of thought and action and difficulty with sequencing and logic. When closely observed the reason for her errors and failures was seen to be consistently due to the fact that she was still answering or responding to a question or task that she had understood a few minutes previously.

Like a needle in the old-fashioned gramophone she had got stuck in a groove! Staff had to remember what had occurred as long as 30 minutes ago before they understood her remarks.

Under these circumstances any long explanation was inappropriate. She was incapable of responding to any stratagem. Hyperventilation was also quite obviously occurring, as whenever she perceived even minor pressures she began to breathe so fast that she made a series of gasping sounds. When these were timed the rate was estimated at about 30 breaths a minute.

A simple, staged intervention was planned. Only that part immediately concerned with HV will be outlined here.

Mr A's co-operation was sought and an attempt was made to slow her breathing rate and to encourage a more shallow level. The system of counting '1000, 2000' was tried, but owing to the receptive difficulties, as could be expected, this proved a total failure. Mr A, who was in his late 70s and rather impatient, was not able to help very much either. Further thought was given to the implications of the frontal impairments, and another programme was introduced.

Distraction, by the use of rhythm, as used in melodic intonation therapy (Sparks and Holland, 1976) had proved useful in improving Mrs A's communication skills. The value of distraction in frontal cases has been shown in rehabilitation programmes (see Chapter 8). All the usual procedures for retraining HV problems were abandoned. Observations were made on the kind of situations which provoked Mrs A's HV. They always occurred when she was under pressure, or became angry. Distraction was introduced. Every time she began to breathe more fiercely very simple distractors were employed: 'Oh look, aren't those nice flowers?' or 'Have you had your hair done, it looks nice?', are examples. Gesture accompanied the comment in order to assist understanding. Mr A found this easy to do, and all staff consistently followed this policy. HV disappeared remarkably quickly. After three months HV was no longer a problem.

Case 2

Mr T was an apparently fit, healthy and active 82-year-old. As a result of his wife's dramatic and colourful accounts of his strange behaviour a full medical investigation was carried out. Nothing was found. Mrs T had a history of osteoarthritis and was undoubtedly prone to gross exaggerations. When a psychological appraisal was made it became obvious that there was a marital problem of many years duration. Mr T did exhibit restless, rather anxious behaviour, and occasionally had dizzy spells when out, but Mrs T appeared the more emotionally disturbed. The situation was somewhat akin to a folie-à-deux. Interviews were extremely difficult as each partner insisted on expressing strong views about the other, and both were suspicious of leaving the other alone with the psychologist — in fact the one 'outside' would listen at the door! The subject of illness dominated all Mrs T's contributions to the discussions.

Their home was attractive and immaculately maintained. They had many opportunities for outings and holidays, and sufficient capital for them to lead a comfortable existence. The vicious circle had been set up in the early days of marriage and a strategy to turn attention away from finding fault towards mutual help in enjoying life was indicated. Also the gasping and sighing from both parties during interviews required closer consideration.

Both partners, in a joint session, were asked to count their breath rate. Each had a rate of over 24 breaths a minute. Both claimed to have noticed the other's heavy breathing at certain times during the day. The pretty living room had a large wall clock with a clear second hand. The couple were taught to use the 'second hand' strategy, to sit down together, at least once a day, regularly and practise breath control. They were also to do this before going out, before doing something strenuous or before becoming involved in something potentially anxiety-provoking. The session should last for about ten minutes.

The couple found this easy to do. They quite enjoyed the idea of having something that they could tell the other to do. Their progress was monitored over a two-month period and they developed a routine which was apparently effective. Mrs T certainly resented the negative response to her outbursts about her husband, but she stopped complaining. She also admitted that he had improved; she even stated that her pains were less of a problem. It was highly unlikely that all would be sweet peace, but they spent the following summer going out and about and actually enjoyed themselves. After six months no further cries for help were heard.

Case 3

Mrs P, a lady of 68 years, had been attending a neurological outpatient clinic for some years. She had a history of migraine and more recently of dizzy spells, falls and palpitations. Epilepsy, amongst other possibilities, had been considered. She was a widow, and though her family lived fairly near, she had maintained her own home, elegant way of life and independence. She was cultured, intelligent and socially active.

In view of her falls she became increasingly anxious about crossing roads and worried about possible difficulties arising when she went out. Although she persisted in going out despite her fears, she complained of acute chest discomfort and palpitations when faced with the need to cross a road. Tranquillizers were prescribed some years previously, but the neurologists were unwilling to increase medication and suspected that HV played a major role in the situation.

Because she was so able the usual muscle relaxation strategy was the intervention of choice. She practised this religiously. However, she continued to have panics at roadsides as she found it hard to generalise the relaxation technique to specific difficulties. She also found it hard to accept that HV was the root cause of the symptoms.

The HPT (hyperventilation provocation test) was used with care and for only 30 seconds. In that time her symptoms were clearly precipitated, and it was necessary for her to exhale and reinhale from a paper bag for a little while in order to recover. She found this experience impressive, and discussed the implications. She was taught how to breathe more slowly and given a handout of instructions. The relaxation tape was extended to include the breathing exercises. Her progress was regularly monitored over several months. She learned to use easy breathing in tense situations very quickly, and found it helpful. She continued to need support and encouragement, but on an increasingly longer interval. She was able to cut down the use of tranquillizers and the feeling of self-control over the symptoms gave her increasing confidence. She even managed to sell her home and buy another, with the minimum of help and without any form of panic.

FINAL COMMENTS

Although it is advisable to examine fully the physiological changes in order to establish that HV really is the cause of the client's difficulties, it is not always a suitable procedure to adopt with the elderly. Often the presence of increased rates of breathing can be subjectively established and an appropriate intervention provided which will at least allow the individual the opportunity to exercise some control over his or her life. Often the elderly are concerned about having a stroke or a heart attack, or become anxious about day-to-day difficulties. Such stress can provoke symptoms which appear to be, or are interpreted as being, of a serious nature. To provide the client with reassurance is important, but it is equally important to provide the person with a convincing strategy that can be employed to assist them and to rebuild confidence.

Panic attacks are common problems in general practice and in care situations. General practitioners and staff in hospitals and residential homes could also benefit from knowledge of these simple procedures to help their clients. In many anxiety-provoking situations adults have been taught to use relaxation tapes so that they can develop their own coping skills. The use of tranquillizers may prove efficacious in some instances, but it is always more satisfactory to teach a person to help himself or herself. With the elderly it is necessary to look at the needs of each individual and to tailor the interventions to those needs. The use of HV techniques provides yet another opportunity to preserve a client's independence and to extend rather than limit control over his or her pattern of living and behaving.

REFERENCES

Bass, C. and Gardner, W.N. (1985a) Emotional influences on breathing and breathlessness. *Journal of Psychosomatic Research, 29,* 599–609

Bass, C. and Gardner, W.N. (1985b) Respiratory and psychiatric abnormalities in chronic symptomatic hyperventilation. *British Medical Journal, 290,* 1387–90

Cannon, W.B. (1920) *Bodily changes in pain, hunger, fear and rage,* 2nd edn. Appleton, New York

Clark, D.M., Salkovskis, P.M. and Chalkley, A.J. (1985) Respiratory control as a treatment for panic attacks. *Journal of Behaviour*

Therapy and Experimental Psychiatry, 16, 23–30

Du Laurens, A. (1559) 'A discourse of the preservation of the sight; of melancholke disease; of rheumes and of old age'. London

Haldane, J.S. and Poulton, E.P. (1908) The effects of want of oxygen on respiration. *Journal of Physiology, 37*, 390

Kartsounis, L.D. (1987) Hyperventilation and its relationship with anxiety: a review. Unpublished

Kartsounis, L.D. and Turpin, G. (1987) Effects of induced hyperventilation on electrodermal response habituation to agoraphobia — relevant stimuli. *Journal of Psychosomatic Research, 31*, 401–12

Lum, L.C. (1975) Hyperventilation: the tip and the iceberg. *Journal of Psychosomatic Research, 19*, 375–83

Lum, L.C. (1977) Hyperventilation, *Chest, Heart and Stroke Journal, 2*(1), 7–12

Lum, L.C. (1981) Hyperventilation and anxiety state. *Journal of the Royal Society of Medicine, 74*, 1–4

McKell, T.E. and Sullivan, A.J. (1947) The hyperventilation syndrome in gastroenterology. *Gastroenterology, 9*, 6–18

Pfeffer, J.M. (1978) The aetiology of the hyperventilation syndrome. *Psychotherapy and Psychosomatics, 30*, 47–55

Sparks, R. and Holland, A.L. (1976) Melodic intonation therapy for aphasia. *Journal of Speech and Hearing Disorders, 41*, 287–97

Wood, P. (1941) Hyperventilation. *British Medical Journal, 1*, 805

8

Management, Rehabilitation and Retraining

Una Holden

There are well established principles and strategies that can be incorporated into our programmes ... positive reinforcement, extinction, shaping ... teaching techniques from mental handicap, reality orientation from geriatrics ... and the individual approach from neuropsychology (Wilson, 1981).

CRITICAL ISSUES

Part of the role of a neuropsychologist is the responsibility for developing rehabilitation and retraining programmes, evaluating them and providing evidence to show their effectiveness. Unfortunately, until recently there has been more concern about identifying the nature of disorders than in providing answers or programmes to overcome or alleviate them. Within the past ten years more emphasis has been laid on this important aspect of care. However, the number of satisfactory interventions or rehabilitative measures that have been published is disappointing (Miller, 1984) and there remains a great need for more studies and accepted methods for use with clients who have suffered some form of brain damage. As there is a paucity of approaches for the younger population it is hardly surprising to find that guidelines for use with the over-60s are almost non-existent. This does not mean that in clinical practice nothing at all is being offered as rehabilitation for the elderly. A variety of approaches, methods and techniques are in operation, and some of these will be outlined in this chapter. It is the lack of evaluation studies and the limited range of such interventions, not to mention the general unawareness of them, that require further consideration.

Physiotherapists, occupational therapists and speech therapists all have special approaches in daily use. However, most disciplines work in isolation from each other and there is a reluctance or a difficulty in developing a team system where the different methods can be slotted together into a more meaningful whole.

Goal setting is very loose and poorly organised. The nursing process has much to recommend it, but on many occasions the targets are stated in a negative manner and set at impossible levels. If a group of specialists could sit together and discuss a case it would be simpler for each one to provide the appropriate input to a particular priority. An awareness of the roles of others can limit unnecessary overlap or even contradiction. It can also minimise the degree of confusion for the client caused by the various instructions and multiplicity of strange faces. The policy of alternative methods is outmoded, and the parallel approach is to be preferred (Verwoerdt, 1981).

Common sense in management is often neglected. To fail to recognise the feelings and fears of both client and family could lead to further complications, poor expectations and unwanted stress. It is vital to focus on the individual — his or her needs, interests, abilities and standards of living — as such information can form the basis of most interventions, as well as providing further insight into the nature of the person's difficulties.

Management

The main considerations here should be:

1. counselling, both client and relative;
2. common-sense approaches;
3. the understanding by staff;
4. a search for retained abilities;
5. goal setting and the parallel intervention policy.

Counselling

Fears and anxieties naturally arise when problems occur. Many clients have insight into their difficulties and are afraid of the future. Relatives experience great anxiety, as they have no idea what the future might hold for them or for the changing person who they have known for so long. The need for some explanation is great; in most cases the need to do something is equally great. It is desirable to provide the client and relatives with something positive.

Before any investigations begin the client should be informed, gently, that everyone is trying to help, that they are examining every angle in order to do this and that they understand how upsetting such investigations can be. If the client is at ease with the staff then it is possible to minimise the effects of anxiety. If a similar explanation is given to the relatives it will be easier to judge how involved they wish to be, or can be. If, as is usually the case, they want to help and require guidance, then it is possible to promise to provide guidelines as soon as relevant interventions are planned. Simple interim guidelines and advice should be offered at this early stage. The person could be encouraged to do as much for himself or herself as possible; confidence can be built up by encouragement, by pointing out all the things that *can* be done, and the retained abilities and skills that have been in use without the person being fully aware of them.

With specific disorders immediate aid might include medication, special exercises or encouragement to continue particular pursuits. Instead of hiding away from friends contact should be maintained. The family, instead of taking over completely, could support the person and reinforce all efforts at self-care. If the problem concerns subcortical states the use of the word 'dementia' could lead to inaccurate beliefs and poor expectations. For instance, because the person is slow to respond, others assume that a response is not possible. If both client and relatives know that patience and encouragement will elicit a response the person will make better attempts to do so.

Early stages are important in setting expectations, and every effort should be made to provide support for all concerned. The role of the family will be discussed further later in this chapter.

Common-sense approaches

Many problems can be solved by considering what the obvious solution might be. If it is not possible to identify areas in a building there is probably a lack of signs or information, so the 'disoriented' person may be exhibiting normal behaviour. The inability of most hospitalised patients to know the day or date may be due to the lack of calendars that can be seen or read; there is rarely a reason to distinguish one day from another in most institutions. If someone else appears responsible for doing all the chores it soon becomes easier to leave them to it. If a person is left alone for hours on end, if no explanation is offered for interference in personal privacy, and personal contact and concern are lacking it is hardly surprising that depressions, withdrawal and institutionalisation occur.

Common sense would indicate that if strange behaviours occur that have not been present previously, careful investigations are required. The wish to live, despite disabilities, is accompanied by some degree of motivation, and in order to have motivation there is a need to have a reason for living. In everyday situations people discourage or reinforce the behaviour of others. The comedian who persists in telling a joke at which no-one laughs will not proceed very far in the profession. A person makes friends with others by responding with warmth to those whose company is sought. Such commonplace day-to-day strategies, once they are given a term such as 'behaviour modification', become shrouded in mysticism! What was a routine response suddenly becomes very complicated, and carers appear to experience great difficulty in using such a natural response with clients. The simple solution of not giving too much attention to a child's minor injury, distracting him or her by reinforcing coping skills so that he or she can forget about it quickly, is forgotten when the situation involves an elderly adult demanding attention for a variety of unimportant reasons.

So many of the problems encountered in the home, residential accommodation and hospital fall into this category, and yet the obvious response is rarely perceived. Most of the problems unrelated to brain dysfunction can be changed by ignoring the aberrant behaviours and reinforcing the acceptable, normal ones. Even in the management and rehabilitation of clients with specific impairments reinforcement and modification have a major role to play. Praising and encouraging self-care attempts, or any evidence of ability, will have an effect on motivation and an increase in the individual's wish to live.

It is also sensible to consider what is being offered in the environment by way of inducements to improve. If the atmosphere is sterile, limiting and far removed from normal living then, obviously, motivation cannot blossom. Monitoring of behaviour can lead to the individual being forced into a pattern of behaviour that causes staff no problem, but completely submerges the individual. The environment *must* be active, helpful, interesting and provide opportunities to continue normal living patterns for each individual. Each individual should be able to exercise some control over such an environment.

Search for retained abilities

Very few elderly people with cognitive impairments are globally damaged. The area of retained ability may be small and well hidden, but even an individual who has sustained severe damage will be capable of doing something reasonably well. It is important to identify such abilities as soon as possible (see Chapter 2). By using retained function it is possible to set realistic goals and build up an appropriate rehabilitation programme. If cognitive, daily living and neuropsychological abilities, as well as social factors, are not clear the goals and programmes will be in jeopardy and may well fail.

Goal setting

After assessments are complete and priorities have been established by the team, realistic goals can be set (Barraclough and Fleming, 1985). Goals should be positive, achievable and simple. It is easier to set a new goal at a higher level than attempt to recover the loss caused by setting goals too high. As discussed in Chapter 2 targets must be clearly stated, taking all aspects into consideration and not seeking the impossible. They should be staged, recorded and the person's wishes and priorities should be included. Goals should extend the person's behaviours rather than limit them, and he or she should be involved in setting up the programme.

Some of the targets might well include retraining of lost abilities, e.g. communication, perception. The target must be reasonable and take into account the degree of severity of the damage for such targets to be realistic.

The parallel approach

This concerns the planning stage of goal setting where priorities are considered and the professionals concerned decide where each can be of most help. Co-ordination of services, particular responsibilities and monitoring can be achieved this way. Here it is possible to ensure that available assistance will not prove overwhelming and inappropriate.

REHABILITATION AND RETRAINING

Alzheimer's disease and MID or strokes

Ideally interventions for a client suffering from suspected Alzheimer's disease should commence as soon as possible. Unfortunately, it is usually some time before help is sought or made available.

Essentially, confidence rebuilding is the first step — as it is with most patients. Retained abilities must be highlighted, staff and friends can encourage independence and self-care as much as possible. Simple measures for combating memory loss can be introduced. Conversations can be used to provide each individual with an opportunity to contribute something from his or her knowledge and experience. Well-learned material, responses to familiar situations and places will help the person to behave with confidence. It is new material or experiences which provoke anxiety and error.

The environment is another important factor. Familiar surroundings can usually be the easiest to recognise and help to put the person at ease. Familiar faces, places and situations are more meaningful and supportive. Day-to-day habits, likes, dislikes and routines play major roles in this. Change can prove catastrophic. Taking the individual on a holiday to a strange place, moving him or her from one home to another, or decorating and 'modernising' the home will only add to the confusion. Patience with early word-finding and memory difficulties will lessen the stress of the insightful individuals.

Families, and carers generally, should avoid over-protectiveness, or treating an adult like a child. To remove a person's right to care for himself or herself by washing, dressing or feeding him or her can only lead to greater dependency and an increase of stress for all concerned. There *may* come a time when this might prove necessary, but it is unwise and improper to ensure that it does. The longer a person retains self-responsibility the longer independence and self-interest will be preserved.

Day-to-day skills — washing, washing-up, putting away, bed-making, dusting, etc. — are well-learned skills, but they are boring! Each individual has special interests and retained skills; these too can be used to combat intellectual decline and the pleasant aspect of such activities requires emphasis. If Mr Smith went regularly for a drink with his friends at the local pub he should be encouraged to continue to do so. Perhaps his friends might need to give him a little support, but friends are usually happy to do anything they can to help.

In care situations, when the disease process is more advanced, or appears to be, normal living patterns and self-care remain of paramount importance. Here environmental considerations are prominent (Holden, 1984). An unhelpful or totally undemanding environment can accelerate impairments and decline. The simple rules to establish a good environment are:

Provide private, recognisable space.
Provide active, interesting and easily identifiable public space.
Ensure that important areas are identifiable.
Ensure that opportunities for self-care and daily living skills are available.
Ensure that the individual has reasonable control over the environment.
Ensure that there are opportunities to continue social contact and develop a group identity.
Ensure that relevant information is readily available — time, date, events and news, etc.

The use of reality orientation (Holden and Woods, 1988); reminiscence (Norris, 1986; Coleman, 1986); group living (Rothwell, Britton and Woods, 1983; Booth and Phillips, 1987); and the various exercise, music, drama and movement therapies, plus other approaches, are relevant aids to memory, orientation and the maintenance of abilities, skills and sociability. They may also make some impact on the level of dementia (Charatan, 1984).

RO (reality orientation) can be used in individual programmes for specific problems (Hanley and Gilhooly, 1986; Holden and Woods, 1988). Clients who only attend a day centre or hospital one or more times a week have benefited from verbal RO retraining (Greene, Timbury, Smith and Gardiner, 1983).

MID. Here it is even more vital to identify retained abilities. The shock and distress of both patient and relatives require calming and minimising before rehabilitative programmes can commence. It is necessary to ascertain the condition of language and perception as interventions will be focused accordingly. If language impairments are present it will be necessary to improve communication by the use of pictorial material. If spatial and perceptual difficulties are the main result of the vascular accident then language can remain the main medium for retraining.

Although many adults and children recover from a stroke, a number of staff members, as well as the general public, are under the impression that a stroke in old age will lead to permanent damage of a severe nature. In training, and in discussions with clients and relatives, it is important to point out, if necessary, that many older people also recover and continue normal living. The person's future is in jeopardy if no-one believes that normal recovery is possible. Long-term hospitalisation or continual care will involve clients who have sustained more severe strokes or series of strokes causing numerous deficits which interfere with the individual's capacity to cope with independent living.

It is not always easy to identify those functions which are retained or which are temporarily out of action. It may well require a great deal of patient observation and enquiry, and considerable effort, to elicit co-operation from the client. The hardest thing for a therapist to accept is a client's refusal to co-operate. If motivation cannot be aroused, if the person clearly chooses to withdraw, to make no attempt to improve functioning or even chooses to die, then there is nothing that anyone can do to force events to change. An individual has the right to choose and no-one can interfere with that choice. Alternatives can be made obvious, and the individual should be given the opportunity to consider them, but in the end it is that person who makes the decision. All staff can do in these circumstances is to provide warmth, good care and much patience — the person may change his or her mind. Staff need to give each other support and feel free to talk about the situation. Feelings of guilt and inadequacy are not appropriate, but do need open discussions.

Details about specific deficits and their management or treatment will be discussed below.

Subcortical states

These are fully described in Chapter 4.

Obviously each disorder poses different problems and requires a slightly different approach. Each individual will be different and have different needs and priorities. There are, however, a few general points to be considered:

1. The patient retains intellectual abilities until late in the course of the condition.
2. Slow, or even lack of, response does not signify an inability to respond or a lack of motivation.
3. If the reactions of others are impatience, irritability or dismissal the patient will become withdrawn, depressed or even despairing.
4. If distractions or ways to split concentration on a task are employed the patient can usually respond more easily.
5. Intensive research continues to look for techniques to assist these patients and to increase understanding of the disease process.
6. Drug therapies are also being developed.

Encouragement, understanding, giving more time, and reinforcing responses can be of considerable assistance to the person.

Family and friends

In order to provide support for families information on relevant societies and associations can be made available. Help is offered in many ways, and from a variety of sources. In Great Britain there are many national organisations as well as local ones, e.g. Age Concern, Help the Aged, the Alzheimer's Society, Parkinson's Association, Headway, etc. *The 36 Hour Day* is a useful reference for these addresses (Mace, Rabins, Castleton, Cloke and McEwen, 1985). Relatives support groups and stroke clubs operate in many cities and towns throughout the country. Usually they are attached to hospitals or centres for the elderly, neurological or head injury units. Information can be obtained via the hospital in each locality, probably through the occupational or speech therapy departments. Relatives and clients can be offered guidance and help, not only through the relevant medical department, but also by clinical psychology.

It is often of value to supply relatives or clients with written guidelines, as it is so easy to forget all the advice that has been provided in an interview (Church, 1983). Any handout should be checked to ascertain that it is relevant to the needs of the client, and efforts should be made to tailor it accordingly. The suggested guidelines in Appendices 1 and 2 will not be suitable for every individual. The person could be functioning at a very high level or at a poor one, so it is necessary to pick out the ideas relevant to that situation, or to produce a totally new set of guidelines. Packages can be taken as law!

To suggest to a poorly paid family that they are required to spend large sums of money on electronic games would be unrealistic. However, there are many games on the market which can make relearning a pleasure and something all the family can join in on. Some of them are electronic and some of them are fairly reasonably priced items that might be bought for family amusement, but they are also geared to using specific skills such as memory, hand–eye co-ordination, spatial perception and the use of language. If a person has only minimum deficits and is of a high intellectual level something more stimulating than household chores is required to increase motivation. To aid language skills games such as Scrabble, Lexicon cards, and other word games can prove invaluable. Spatial problems can benefit from three-dimensional games such as Connect 4, Spacelines, Trac 4, mosaics, jigsaws and so forth. There is a wide range of game-like aids for memory including the electronic ones, e.g. Adam, Wizard and Simon. On a simpler level shopping lists, prices, calculation of bills and the use of diaries can be recommended. With the help of relatives a person could make notes on an interesting item of news on the radio and follow it up during the day. Newspapers and television could add another angle on the same item, and the family could ask the person if he or she can remember the information without notes, or with them if problems occur.

More severely impaired clients living at home would need more simple reminders. Relatives could use The 24 Hour Approach (Holden, White and Martin, 1979) which provides suggestions on how to use simple RO, the use of the past tense and how to ensure that the environment is helpful. Calendars, reminder boards and diaries are all relevant. Verbal RO stresses the use of tenses, positive statements, short sentences, one concept at a time to avoid confusion and the use of repetition to aid memory.

'That's right Dad, you *used* to ... didn't you?'

This is preferable to a head-on confrontation about mixing the present with the past.

'It *was* good when Dad was here, I know you miss him'.

This will avoid repeating the information that Dad died years ago. 'You did that well' is more positive and encouraging than 'You are doing better' or 'you can do better'.

'Would you like to wear the pink jumper?' is easier to answer than 'Would you prefer the green or the pink jumper?' Repetitions do not need to be parrot-like. 'It's time to get up, Mum' could be followed by 'Breakfast is ready, are you nearly dressed?' Information can be imparted again and again without actually repeating the same words. This allows the person time to grasp the necessary concept, and helps relatives to avoid the frustration caused by saying the same thing over and over again.

SPECIFIC DEFICITS

'Remediating cognitive deficit remains the greatest challenge to those concerned with the rehabilitation of the brain-injured' (Diller, 1976). Rehabilitation sessions should be short, frequent, interesting to the client and require plenty of praise and encouragement.

Orientation and attention

Many confused old people ramble, talk about irrelevant subjects and do not appear to answer questions sensibly. A simple remedy is to use good eye contact, slow speech and gentle touch on a hand or on an arm. If the question is put clearly in this way an appropriate response will probably be made. The length of time that normal attention lasts will vary, and the strategy will have to be employed again. However, if this occurs regularly the person is given practice in attending, and the span will lengthen.

Time sense can be assisted by a large, clear clock placed where it can be seen. If staff point it out and regularly ask the person to tell the time he or she will learn to look without help.

Calendars and notice-boards can be used to highlight specific information such as holidays, special events, mealtimes and favourite television programmes.

Orientation with regard to place can be improved by signs and notices, pictures, photographs, maps and views from a window. All these might be available, but clients require constant reminders to use or notice them.

Orientation concerning person can be helped by the use of photographs, pictures, magazines, television and even mirrors.

Aphasias

Language disorders are described in detail in Chapter 5. Here, several points are relevant. If language skills are intact they are available for use in rehabilitation programmes. The person will be capable of expressing ideas and fears by both spoken and written words. Understanding of the language of others, both spoken and written, will also be intact, or reasonably so. Therefore instructions, suggestions and other information can be written down and the whole field of communication is available to the therapist even though, in some instances, thoughts and responses may be a little confused.

If language is impaired there are multiple effects:

Social contacts and outlets are limited.
Understanding of and by a person is limited.
Other methods of communication are required.
Relatives and staff can overlook the individual personality
    and see the person as a being in need of total care.
Basic intelligence is assumed to be lost.

So it is essential to:

1. Help others to appreciate the hidden intelligence and the individual.
2. Speak slowly, clearly and simply to aid understanding.
3. Explain any intervention.
4. Give the person time to comprehend or to respond.
5. Use other means of communication, e.g. gesture, pictures, writing, letters or matching. Speech may improve, perhaps only one word at a time.

6. Use retained and spatial abilities. When the person picks up an object provide a picture of it too. Say the name and encourage the client to say it too. If prompting words does not work, then do not persist immediately, just use pictures to communicate.

Several manuals on helping speech problems have been published (e.g. Fawcus, Robinson, Williams and Williams, 1983) and can provide useful ideas for both individual and group work.

Apraxias

Rehabilitation studies have been chiefly concerned with aphasias and this disorder of movement has been badly neglected. A recent book by Miller (1986) gathers together most of the relevant information, theory and some guidelines on the subject but more good treatment programmes are still required. Luria (1963) provided a number of examples of retraining programmes, but there has been little or no attempt to replicate or evaluate his work. Here some simple ideas which have proved of use in clinical practice will be outlined, but it must be stressed that they may not be of value in every case.

If the person is very disabled it is difficult to assess the presence of an apraxia, particularly if there is a post-trauma weakness of the limbs or hands.

Peripheral weakness or residual lack of full control can be helped by graded exercises or interesting tasks. A miniature piano can be used to improve the strength of fingers. For the same purpose stacking plastic or paper cups, sorting buttons into sets or cutting out pictures or materials for a collage can be meaningful ways of exercising the hands and fingers. Those with a slight apraxia might also benefit from these activities, though some guiding of the hands or modelling will be required before the person can get started.

Putting words and pictures together can be helpful. For example a series of pictures with stage-by-stage instructions on how to shave, how to put on lipstick, or how to make a sandwich, can help an apraxic person complete a task. This will split concentration between performing the action and following the instructions. As there is an appropriate verbal message on each picture the presence or absence of language disability is not a problem. As *distraction* is the important element in retraining apraxic individuals the mixture of picture and words can prove effective too.

Melodic intonation therapy (Sparks and Holland, 1976) has been used as a treatment with certain types of aphasia. Rhythm, music and beat have a use with movement disorders too. It is vital to avoid giving an apraxic patient direct instructions or orders about performing a task or action. To tell such a person to 'Brush your teeth' or 'pick up your fork and knife' will almost certainly lead to a failure. However, if the person is encouraged to sing or hum a tune to himself or herself at the same time as the action is to be performed, success is more likely to occur. Another person can do the singing, humming or time beating, but in due course the person should learn to do this alone. To the chant of 'up and down, up and down' the person may giggle but teeth get cleaned! Having more than one action or idea to consider removes the degree of voluntary focus on the required action.

The rigid clenching of fists resulting from a conscious attempt to perform a task can be relaxed by a change of conversation or a diversion of attention. Relatives and staff would find it more productive to talk about the look and smell of food, or even the state of the weather, than to give an apraxic person direct instructions on how to eat the food.

Sometimes actually miming an action will spark off the correct response; demonstrating with actual objects can also help. A touch of humour can prove invaluable as a distraction.

Dressing apraxia. This difficulty in dressing can be caused by many different impairments and there are variations from individual to individual. It will be necessary to try a number of strategies before an effective method can be found, for example:

> *Colour* — Red tabs on the back of clothes. A yellow tab with *left* for the left shoe, and a green tab with *right* for the right shoe.
> *Order* — Laying out clothes in the order in which that particular individual usually dresses.
> *Spoken instruction, with a guiding hand* — Talk through each stage while using a prompting gesture. Start the person off, then allow him or her to finish putting on each item.

Mime — Pretend to put on an item.
Demonstrate — actually put on, or start to put on an item, then hand it to the person.

Aims should be low at first, allowing the person to do as much alone as possible, giving lots of time and working step by step.

Praise and encouragement are given at each little success. This may take time until some progress is made, but it is better to take some time to find a solution than to continually spend time dressing and undressing the person on a daily basis.

Spatial disorders

Losing the way, even in familiar places, can cause frustration and anxieties not only for relatives and staff but also for the person. In severe cases the starting point could be the drawing of rooms and using cut-outs of relevant pieces of furniture and equipment. The patient could be asked to put together a kitchen, sitting room or bedroom, placing the pieces of furniture in the appropriate places. When this is done he or she could be asked 'Is this like your room at home?'

Attempts to replicate the organisation of rooms at home could form the next stage. He or she can be asked to describe:

'How do you find your way to your bedroom/living room/ bathroom etc?'
'What are the colours of the walls and carpets in ...?'
'What materials/textures are used for curtains/furnishings?'
'What style/shape is your furniture in ...?'

This can provoke associations and help the person to recall forgotten clues. At a later stage drawing maps at increasing levels of difficulty could be tried:

The street on which he or she lives.
The main shopping street, with the supermarket, chemist, newsagent, etc. Here real photographs can be used which will make the exercise more realistic and interesting.
Larger maps of the entire country can be introduced and major towns and places identified.

The use of coloured lines along walls to the toilet can be used at home as well as in institutions, and has been shown to cut down the incidence of 'accidents'. Patterns and colours on doors can make identification easier.

Orientation is improved by signs — both picture and word — and familiar pictures or objects hung on or by the door of a person's room can improve ability to identify private space.

If a residential home or ward has clues to the whereabouts of areas and important places clients can be taught to find their own way by regular, guided tours. The clues are pointed out again and again, and then each client acts as the guide showing staff around (Hanley, 1981). Orientation, to the situation at least, is improved.

Confusion at home can be aided by the use of little pictures and words placed in relevant positions. Cutlery, clothing, linen and jewellery, for example, can all be found and replaced if the person has a clue to identify where things go. As in ward training, constant reminders about the clues will be necessary at first. With clients living alone, home organisers, or visiting nursing staff, could act as guides and reinforcers until a routine is established.

The useful shop games in which space plays a part can be of value here. Spacelines, Connect 4, Trac 4, etc., are all relevant. Painting, drawing and cutting out to make collages will provide more practice at handling spatial tasks.

Agnosias

Some of the few attempts to retrain patients with agnosias have been outlined by Miller (1984). Luria (1963) had a particular interest in agnostic problems, but his clients were mainly younger wounded soldiers, and the single case reports are not always relevant to the problems of the elderly with agnosic difficulties.

Perceptual errors can prove confusing and anxiety-provoking for both client and relative. The solution to most object agnosias is really quite simple, though it may not always be effective as other problems might be involved. Usually if the person is encouraged to use other senses as well recognition will occur. Sight alone will not help but the touch, taste and smell — as appropriate — will hasten normal identification. Other forms of agnosia will also benefit from the use of a number of senses. Touch might require sight or smell, smell might require visual confirmation. *Auditory agnosia* is slightly different. If the difficulty is with understanding the spoken words of other people, slower speech on their part can remove the difficulty. The person appears unable to cope with the normal rate of speech, but once it is slowed down he or she experiences no lack of comprehension. Agnosia for non-verbal sounds can be dangerous as the person needs to see the source of the noise before being able to identify it. It is unfortunate that barking, angry dogs cannot be persuaded to bark more slowly, and it is impossible to influence the rate of noise made by objects so this form of agnosia remains a problem.

Body image disturbances. These are usually short-lived in the acute form. Neglect of one side can be helped by common-sense strategies. Turn the plate around when the person eats the side within his or her vision. Place beds so that the person can see the way to and from the toilet. Talk and work with the client from the side to which he or she responds. Explain the situation to staff and family so that they can help and understand.

To encourage response to the neglected side others can make progressive moves from the edge of vision into the neglected area to widen the range of attention. Gently moving the person's head can also help. With reading another strategy is possible.

Place a flat, wide, coloured stick on the edge of the words that can be read in a magazine. Ask the person if he or she can see from that point. When the actual starting point is identified, ask the person to start reading. After a few sentences, distract the attention by remarking on something well inside the area of vision — to the non-neglected side. After a few seconds, during which the stick has been very slightly moved in the other direction, ask the person to recommence reading 'from the edge of the stick as before'. It is possible to extend the field of vision very slowly in this way.

Prosopagnosia and *simultanagnosia* are both still extremely hard to treat. With the former many strategies are required as there is probably an element of psychopathology in some cases. Body image disturbances may respond if the person is required to touch his or her own nose, cheek, hair, etc., while looking in the mirror. The use of photographs, matching, and the sound of familiar voices with 'forgotten' faces can be a help in many instances. Both these disabilities require much further investigation, and as the number of cases is so limited it remains very difficult to find easy answers.

Memory

Like the aphasias memory is seen as a major problem, and as a result has received more attention than some other disabilities. Theoretical aspects have received the greatest input and those readers interested in the mechanisms involved, the areas of the brain that may be concerned and impairments that might result from various lesions or disease processes should consult textbooks on the subject, such as Hecaen and Albert (1978), Poon (1980), Wilson and Moffat (1984), or Woods and Britton (1985).

Miller (1984) provides a useful review of the literature on memory disorders and a critique of methods used to improve them. His conclusion that there is as yet little evidence to show proven effectiveness of clinical measures may be discouraging, but attempts to find answers will, hopefully, eventually identify some relevant strategies. With the elderly even small improvements are welcome, and the reasons for decline in function are so varied that it remains essential to consider the individual rather than memory problems in general.

Wilson and Moffat (1984) and their colleagues have produced a useful account of various memory therapies, and include guidelines on setting up and running memory groups which are popular in many units throughout the country. Wilson and Moffat distinguish between such groups run for the elderly complaining of memory loss but without major cognitive impairment and those with some form of dementia. The latter groups are more appropriately helped in an RO group situation, or with special training programmes to meet a specific need. Planned programmes are provided by Hanley and Gilhooly (1986), whose client wanted to remember that her husband had died, and Holden and Woods (1988) describe plans for a lady who lived in a residential home and a man who lived at his own home, both of whom complained that they had problems remembering things.

Although it is extremely difficult to make great strides in improving memory where function has sustained some form of damage, there are ways to help it, and there are cases of pseudo-memory loss. Emotional factors can interfere with a person's concentration and motivation to learn. Depression leads to disinterest, illness to frailty, and expectations to benign forgetfulness. In all cases real memory loss has not been sustained. It is important to distinguish the real from the apparent or anxiety-related memory deficits as soon as possible, so that the right approach can be employed.

Real memory disorders in elderly people can be helped by individual plans accompanied by group situations where well-learned social responses and pleasant situations can stimulate motivation and response. RO and REM (reminiscence) groups have been found most useful here. In Chapter 6 interventions of use in the early stages of recovery from coma or head injury are described. Other simple methods can be used at later stages, and with those suffering from a dementia-related disorder.

Most people take perceptions for granted and do not pay enough attention to ordinary experiences such as noticing the colour of all the neighbours' front doors, the number of steps up to the bedrooms or even the route taken by a driver. In residential homes and hospitals clients should be encouraged to take note of such little cues so that they can learn to find their way around. Staff could point out name badges, colours of different uniforms, signs on doors and so forth. Clients living at home can be encouraged to notice similar things in their environments so that they can remember the cues to help them find their way, instead of relying on the automatic responses that used to allow them to think of something else while they walked to the local grocer's.

Diaries and notebooks are important, but they must be used and not left forgotten in a drawer. Similarly notice-boards at home, or in the care situation, should have updated information and be used regularly. Staff and relatives can ask questions at regular intervals which will encourage the person to take notice and think about what is happening.

'What did you have for breakfast?', 'Who is coming to see you this afternoon?' 'What are you going to watch on television tonight?' and so forth.

As has been suggested before, games of all kinds can make the memory practice more palatable and more fun.

There are a number of external aids which can be used to help (Harris and Morris, 1984); computer aids are being made available, but cooker timers, digital watches and alarm clocks, as well as diaries, notebooks and notice-boards, are all external aids and all have their uses.

A simple timer can be used in a programme which will slowly build up a person's ability to remember to do things at a specific time. It will require help from another person. One or two particular important appointments can be selected — say going to the Day Centre and preparing an evening meal. The timer can be set first thing in the morning, *by the person* with advice of the helper, for five minutes prior to the time to get ready. The timer will act as a prompt to check the time on a clock and to start preparing to go out. The timer must be reset, then and there, to signal the next appointment. Initially this should only include one or two things to be remembered every day. A record should be kept to show progress and to encourage the person. After a succession of achievements the person can try to set the timer alone. It will require some supervision at first, but once a routine can be established the timer can be used for a variety of things to remember.

Community staff can be a considerable help in ensuring that elderly people living at home have reminders and use them. In hospitals or homes the staff can monitor changes and ensure that opportunities and strategies to aid memory are available and are used.

Frontal damage

Some of the problem behaviours associated with frontal damage have been covered elsewhere in this chapter, so only the ones that are particularly common with the elderly, and which cause concern, will be considered here.

Perseveration

The repetition of words, phrases and actions is probably one of the most distressing behaviours. Staff, relatives and other patients or residents find such repetitiveness very hard to tolerate, and it probably plays a part in stress factors for carers. Distraction is probably the most successful methods of managing this problem. However, there are other methods which have been attempted with varying degrees of success. Behavioural techniques can work well. Often the person uses these perseverative phrases when he or she has been left alone for long periods of time, and the irritating words will prompt a response from staff or others. Often it is not a friendly or warm response, but at least it is a response! If several members of staff can be made key workers — to cover all hours of the day — and if all members of staff are aware of the programme, a consistent plan can be drawn up. The person should be given attention when he or she is not repeating the phrase, and ignored when doing so. It is important to inform the person that this is going to happen, and wise to try to tell other residents too. Unfortunately it is the other residents or patients who can cause the failure with this approach, as it is often impossible for them to refrain from abusive responses to the constant parrot talk!

Recording the person and playing the repetition back to him or her has also been attempted, but with little success. Rarely is the voice recognised and the response is often 'For God's sake shut up' from the perseverator himself or herself!

Luria used interruptions with movements in order to prevent this form of perseveration; the same thing can be successfully applied to verbal perseveration. As the irritating phrase, word or sentence begins, some form of distraction should be initiated. According to the situation and the individual concerned a comment, a noise or a touch can be useful. 'Oh, Mrs Blair, have you seen these flowers?' or 'Mr Peters, have you seen this in the newspaper?' are possible comments. The ensuing normal discussion can provide an opportunity to give the person some attention and encouragement so that more acceptable behaviour can be reinforced.

Other occasions might require a loud hand-clap, dropping something noisily, bell-ringing, or something else which will startle the person sufficiently to interrupt the repetition. As soon as attention is caught, and the perseverations cease, time should be spent with the person talking pleasantly. A gentle hand on the person's arm followed by general talk is also effective as a distraction.

Thought can become one-track too. The 'stuck needle' syndrome also responds to distraction. It can become a game with staff to think of something different in order to give the person's thought processes a jerk so that it is possible to ask a question and obtain a sensible reply.

With repeated gesture or movements it is necessary to interrupt completion or continuation of movement by a restraining hand. This should be done just as the gesture commences, and should be accompanied by warmth and interest in the person, including staying to talk for a time.

In most cases it is advisable to check to see just how active the environment is. If nothing is happening stereotyped behaviour is not uncommon. Even unfortunate animals caged up in a zoo display stereotyped behaviour when they are unable to live normally. Any sterile atmosphere can lead to 'neurotic' behaviour, so before any specific intervention is employed with an individual it is important to ascertain if that behaviour is caused by the poverty of the environment rather than damage to that person's brain.

Poor sequencing ability

An impairment in organisation, in putting things into a logical order, is often seen with head-injured clients. It also happens with elderly confused people. Staged practice in ordering things can help a little. Breaking down a task into its component parts and drawing the person's attention to each separate part is one strategy. Sequential pictures, picture stories or cartoons can be useful. It is advisable to start with two pictures at a time, and with simple concepts. Newspaper or comic cartoons can be used. With three items, such as spring, summer and winter, or baby, child and adult, etc., the client can be asked to sort the pictures into a correct order. Later stages could include more complicated cartoons or, for example, the steps in the growth and flowering of a plant, the making of a cake and so forth.

In more active situations the person's ability to dress could be used, or other daily living skills which are preserved, so that order can be demonstrated. The fact that the person *can* put order into practice successfully should be stressed as encouragement.

Emotional lability or inappropriate emotion

Relatives and staff can become upset by a patient who weeps in the middle of a conversation or suddenly begins to laugh for no real reason. Pity and alarm are the usual reactions. Someone in tears is a moving sight, and everyone wishes to provide comfort or relief. Depression is diagnosed, grief about the present situation seems to be indicated, or even bad treatment is suspected. Certain emotional restraints in brain systems could have been affected so the person cannot control these unwelcome outbursts. Sympathy only makes the situation worse. The insightful patient can be embarrassed and ashamed at this lack of control. If other possibilities are ruled out, the problem should be discussed with the person and an explanation provided. Furthermore it helps to control the flowing emotion if onlookers ignore it and talk as though it was not occurring. This is difficult to do, but if comment to the patient must be made, understanding rather than sympathy, or even irritation, should be expressed.

Recording and evaluation

As there is so much variation from individual to individual in the type and degree of dysfunction it is important to record all interventions, their reason, nature and progress. What might be suitable for one may prove useless with another. If, after a reasonable trial period, an approach does not show any improvement in the person's behaviour or problem, then it is time for a team to discuss another kind of intervention. However, as some of the behaviours may be well-established, or because there might be some lack of consistency or interference in the present approach, careful scrutiny of the programme must be made before considering a change.

As there is still a paucity of useful approaches to help neuropsychological deficits in elderly people, careful recording could lead to evaluation studies which would provide more accepted methods for use clinically. In a 'new' field new ideas are required, and once these appear to be useful they require evaluations so that others can use those that show the most promise. The need for such methods is great not only for the young, but also for the older generations.

REFERENCES

Barraclough, C. and Fleming, I. (1985) *Goal setting with elderly people.* Manchester University Press, Manchester

Booth, T. and Phillips, D. (1987) Group living in homes for the elderly: a comparative study of outcome of care. *British Journal of Social Work, 17,* 1–20

Charatan, F.B. (1984) Mental stimulation and deprivation of risk factors in senility. In H. Rothschild (ed.), *Risk factors in senility* Oxford University Press, New York

Church, M. (1983) Psychological therapy with elderly people. *Bulletin of the British Psychological Society, 36*, 110–12

Coleman, P. (1986) *Ageing and reminiscence processes: social and clinical implications.* Wiley, Chichester and New York

Diller, L. (1976) A model for cognitive retraining in rehabilitation. *Clinical Psychologist, 29,* 13–15

Fawcus, M., Robinson, M., Williams, J. and Williams, R. (1983) *Working with dysphasics.* Winslow Press, Oxford

Greene, J.G., Timbury, G.C., Smith, R. and Gardiner, M. (1983) Reality orientation with patients in the community: an empirical evaluation. *Age and Ageing, 12,* 18–43

Hanley, I.G. (1981) The use of signposts and active training to modify ward disorientation in elderly patients. *Journal of Behaviour Therapy and Experimental Psychiatry, 12,* 241–7

Hanley, I.G. and Gilhooly, M. (1986) *Psychological therapies for the elderly.* Croom Helm, London/New York University Press, New York

Harris, J.E. and Morris, P.E. (eds) (1984) *Everyday memory, actions and absentmindedness.* Academic Press, London

Hecaen, H. and Albert, M.L. (1978) *Human neuropsychology.* Wiley, New York

Holden, U.P. (1984) *Thinking it through.* Winslow Press, Bicester.

Holden U.P., White, M. and Martin, C. (1979) *The 24 hour approach,* Winslow Press, Oxford

Holden, U.P. and Woods, R.T. (1982; 2nd edn 1988) *Reality orientation; psychological approaches to the 'confused' elderly.* Churchill Livingstone, Edinburgh

Luria, A.R. (1963) *Restoration of function after brain injury.* Pergamon Press, Oxford

Mace, N.L., Rabins, P.V., Castleton, B., Cloke, C. and McEwen, E. (1985) *The 36 hour day.* Hodder & Stoughton, Sevenoaks and Age Concern England/Johns Hopkins University Press, Baltimore

Miller, E. (1984) *Recovery and management of neuropsychological impairments.* Wiley, Chichester

Miller, N. (1986) *Dyspraxia and its management.* Croom Helm, London/Aspen Publishers, Rockville, Maryland

Norris, A. (1986) *Reminiscence with elderly people.* Winslow Press, Oxford

Poon, I.W. (1980) A systems approach for the assessment and treatment of memory problems. In J. Ferguson and C. Taylor (eds), *Handbook of behavioural medicine. 1: Systems intervention.* Spectrum, New York, pp. 191–212

Rothwell, N., Britton, P.G. and Woods, R.T. (1983) The effects of group living in a residential home for the elderly, *British Journal of Social Work, 13,* 639–43

Sparks, R. and Holland, A.L. (1976) Melodic intonation therapy for aphasia. *Journal of Speech and Hearing Disorders, 41,* 287–97

216

Verwoerdt, A. (1981) Psychotherapy for the elderly. In T. Arie (ed.), *Health care of the elderly*. Croom Helm, London, pp. 118–39

Wilson, B.A. (1981) Cognitive rehabilitation after brain damage. Paper presented at Annual Conference British Psychological Society

Wilson, B.A. and Moffat, N. (1984) *Clinical management of memory problems*. Croom Helm, London/Aspen Publishers, Rockville, Maryland

Woods, R.T. and Britton, P.G. (1985) *Clinical psychology with the elderly*. Croom Helm, London

Appendix 1

Suggested Guidelines for Non-verbal Impairments

Memory

Any form of memory game is useful, e.g. games such as Scrabble, Monopoly, Lexicon cards, etc. If these are too difficult, then grandchildren can play 'I spy', Kim's Game, etc. Adults can help by quizzes and recent news item questions, 'What was the main news on TV or in the newspaper today?', 'Who gave the news? What date was mentioned?' Notebooks and diaries can be used. If major items of news cannot be recalled then if they are recorded in the notebook they can be checked and the person reminded.

A notice or chalk board in the kitchen can be used daily to remind about date, day, and important things like 'turn on dinner at 4 o'clock'. Routine shopping lists can be made and attached to the notice-board for easy finding.

A large, clear calendar is helpful, so is a large-faced clock. Routines to provide consistent clues in the home can be established. Where to store items or find them can become associated with pictures and words stuck on relevant cupboards, doors or drawers — cutlery, linen, clothes, etc. Sometimes electronic games can be provided — Simon, Adam and Wizard are examples of amusing games to assist memory and dexterity.

Problems with movements

Problems are not just with walking but include 'clumsiness' of hand, confusion in making gestures, perhaps having difficulty with buttons. A piano, either toy or real, is useful to exercise fingers; a typewriter achieves the same goal. Stacking paper or plastic cups, sorting buttons — all these are good for hand and finger movement. Bead threading might prove hard, but guiding hands can be a help initially. For less severe difficulties doing the washing up, folding linen, setting tables, using tools, jigsaws and cutting out for collages are all relevant to relearning movements and the use of hands.

Losing the way

Drawing maps of the home, the street outside and the main shopping street. A plan of the home and other areas will be easier if names are given — kitchen, stairs, Waterloo Road, Main Street, Jones' the butcher, etc. Colour can be added to the drawings — pink carpet, green toilet door — whatever is correct for the person's home.

Signs and little notices can be useful at home as well as in hospital. Distinct colour for the toilet door, perhaps even coloured tape along a wall.

The use of pictures with written words can remind the person how to do something and provide the correct order, e.g. stage-by-stage pictures on how to shave, to make a sandwich, cook a meal, etc.

Three-dimensional games such as Spacelines, Connect 4, etc, can prove a means of bringing all the family together to help. This will make it a pleasure to relearn skills, and be less boring than household chores. Mosaics and jigsaws can be used by the person alone.

Perseveration

Sometimes a person will repeat the same phrase or action. He or she cannot help this. However, if some distraction is introduced this repetitiveness can be lessened. Provide something to look at, interrupt the repetition just as it commences by remarking on some event, interest or give the person something nice to look at, touch or smell. To take a hand gently just as a constantly repeated movement begins, and to talk warmly about some occurrence, will discourage the action. It is important to respond to the *lack* of perseveration rather than to the perseveration itself. If the warm response is associated with the undesirable problem then the repetition will probably increase.

Acquired knowledge

Reading and writing should be encouraged. A library can provide large-print books. Magazines are colourful and easy to manage, books with pictures on topics of interest will encourage the use of knowledge and skills. Word games from shops — Lexicon, Scrabble — can help too.

Emotional changes

Occasionally the elderly person shows sudden, unexpected emotional changes. Inappropriate laughing or crying will occur. These could be due to frustration, but more likely these outbursts are due to an inability to control physiological processes, and have nothing to do with real emotion. Carers should not get upset; instead they should gently distract attention and talk through the outburst as though it was not happening. This can assist in stopping it.

Dressing, eating and body image

A common problem is a poor attempt at self-dressing. Putting clothes out in the order in which the person normally dresses is recommended. Marks or tags on the back of clothes, marks inside shoes to denote the left and right, a guiding hand with buttons, will help most people to get started. A staged programme for eating is advised. First give praise for helping to put a spoon in his or her mouth, then praise for putting the spoon to the mouth without help, then for picking up food with a spoon, then only for completing the whole operation with a spoon without help. At this stage relearning how to use a fork and knife can commence. With guidance and praise most people will learn again.

Neglect of, or ignoring, part of the body are not uncommon consequences of a stroke. Simple measures can help. Turn around a half-eaten plate of food so that the other half can be seen. Place furniture so that it is easier to see all important parts of the room. Talk and work with the person on the side that is not neglected or ignored, move slowly, in stages to the other side.

Perceptual errors

If the person has difficulty in recognising objects by one sense alone — usually sight — allow him or her to use other senses too. Objects may not look familiar, but their feel, taste or smell will probably supply enough information to aid normal recognition.

220

Appendix 2

Suggested Guidelines for Communication Problems

These ideas could help when there are particular difficulties with language.

The correct use of words for particular objects, people, etc, may be impaired, and there may also be difficulties with reading and writing. It is important to appreciate that this does not imply that the person's intelligence is totally lost; furthermore, apart from communication it may not be impaired at all.

Communication is a two-way process. Avoid talking about a person as though he or she was not there. Talk *to* him or her; encourage a response. Perhaps the use of gesture, social expressions or a note-pad might be the only possible means of communicating. If so, use patience and understanding, but encourage their use. Make sure attention is real, keep the conversation clear, simple and to the point, avoiding abstract and emotional topics. Talk about definite topics, people he or she knows, about objects, places or events that can be remembered. If there is evidence of growing frustration, leave things alone for a time. If the person attempts to say something, refrain from supplying the necessary word; give clues instead. Sound the beginning of the word or associate the word with a phrase e.g. 'cup of ...' or 'You're hungry so you want your ...'. Otherwise use examples, e.g. 'It has bristles' or 'You clean your teeth with it'.

Talk normally even if response is impossible or withheld. The person will know *how* you react or speak, even if not understanding all that is said. It is important to remember that basic aids such as teeth, hearing aids and glasses need to be clean, in use and in good working order.

Ideas to provide practice with language

Grandchildren can be very helpful. Elderly people do not feel as threatened by playing simple games with children as they would with an adult. Memory and word games will stimulate thought and provide practice in word-finding and usage. 'Fish' with pictures or words, 'Kim's Game' with objects, pictures or words and basic card games, even 'I spy', are all possible games to play. Many Bingo games can be devised which match words to pictures, sentences to pictures, using opposites, occupations, etc. One word or sentence is on the Bingo card, and the matching one is on the card to be drawn out of the pile.

Recall of words can be encouraged by using pictures with large print for words such as 'saucepans', 'cutlery' or 'groceries'. These can be stuck on relevant drawers, or cupboards throughout the house, especially in the person's own room. When an object is used, encourage the use of the correct word, perhaps by repetition; also try to encourage the person to talk about what is happening during routine tasks, e.g. dressing. Items could be named as they are being put on, and the necessary action could be described. Ask the person to say the words, repeat them, say them in unison or say them alone. The association of the action, objects and words related to it and, where possible, the written word, will help understanding of the words being used.

When out, point out the road signs, advertising notices and shop signs. Read them aloud, encourage him or her to read them too. In shops look at labels and prices and see if simple amounts can be added together so that the correct money, or change, can be estimated.

When errors occur correct *gently*, not making failure too obvious, but always praise and reinforce the successes.

Index